Audiovisual Translation
Subtitles and Subtitling

NEW TRENDS IN TRANSLATION STUDIES
Volume 9

Series Editor:
Dr Jorge Díaz Cintas

Advisory Board:
Professor Susan Bassnett McGuire
Dr Lynne Bowker
Professor Frederic Chaume
Professor Aline Remael

PETER LANG
Oxford • Bern • Berlin • Bruxelles • Frankfurt am Main • New York • Wien

Audiovisual Translation
Subtitles and Subtitling

Theory and Practice

Laura Incalcaterra McLoughlin, Marie Biscio
and Máire Áine Ní Mhainnín (eds)

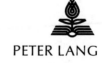

PETER LANG

Oxford • Bern • Berlin • Bruxelles • Frankfurt am Main • New York • Wien

Bibliographic information published by Die Deutsche Nationalbibliothek.
Die Deutsche Nationalbibliothek lists this publication in the Deutsche National-
bibliografie; detailed bibliographic data is available on the Internet at
http://dnb.d-nb.de.

A catalogue record for this book is available from the British Library.

Library of Congress Cataloging-in-Publication Data:

Incalcaterra McLoughlin, Laura.
  Audiovisual translation : subtitles and subtitling : theory and practice / Laura
Incalcaterra McLoughlin, Marie Biscio and Máire Áine Ní Mhainnín.
    p. cm. -- (New trends in Translation studies; 9)
  Includes bibliographical references and index.
  ISBN 978-3-0343-0299-9 (alk. paper)
  1. Translating and interpreting. 2. Mass media and language. 3. Dubbing of mo-
tion pictures. 4. Discourse analysis. 5. Motion pictures--Titling. I. Biscio, Marie.
II. Ní Mhainnín, Máire Áine. III. Title.
  P306.2.M398 2011
  418'.02--dc23
                    2011022533

ISSN 1664-249X
ISBN 978-3-0343-0299-9

© Peter Lang AG, International Academic Publishers, Bern 2011
Hochfeldstrasse 32, CH-3012 Bern, Switzerland
info@peterlang.com, www.peterlang.com, www.peterlang.net

Printed in Germany

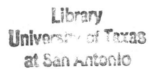

Contents

List of Figures

List of Tables

Acknowledgements

The editors wish to express their gratitude to the IRCHSS – Irish Research Council for the Humanities and Social Sciences – for their generous grant in support of this publication.

We would also like to thank Andrés Zsögön for granting permission to publish a screenshot from DivXLand Media Subtitler.

Introduction

An increasing number of contributions have appeared, over recent years, on the subject of Audiovisual Translation (AVT), particularly in relation to dubbing and subtitling, to the extent that this has become "one of the fastest growing areas in the field of Translation Studies" (Díaz-Cintas, 2008: 1). Many international conferences have been dedicated to this topic and several undergraduate and postgraduate courses have been developed in third level institutions across Europe, some entirely devoted to subtitling and training of subtitlers whilst others use subtitling as an effective pedagogical tool for foreign language (FL) teaching and learning.

The broad scope of this branch of Translation Studies is challenging, an AV text being a truly "multidimensional space" in the sense intended by Barthes (1977: 176), which transcends and links several sensory dimensions. Audiovisual Translation amalgamates diverse disciplines including film studies, translatology, semiotics, linguistics, applied linguistics, cognitive psychology, to name but a few, not forgetting, of course, technology and ICT.

However, as Orero (2004: viii) writes, "though much work has been done over the years by scholars such as Yves Gambier and Henrik Gottlieb, there is still plenty of scope at both academic levels: teaching and researching". This publication is primarily intended for both "academic levels". The first section is dedicated to theoretical issues, which, it is hoped, will stimulate further debate and encourage exciting progress in research informed teaching. The second section lends itself to a perhaps less developed area of research in the field of AVT and its potential in foreign language pedagogy.

The sequence of articles in this volume is intended to create a discourse which, beginning with reflections on wider methodological issues, advances to a proposed model of analysis for colloquial speech, touches on more "niche" aspects of AVT (e.g. surtitling) and progresses to didactic applications in foreign language pedagogy and learning at both linguistic and cultural levels and concludes with a practical proposal for use of AVT in FL classes. An interview with a professional subtitler (who is also an academic and a researcher) draws the volume to a close, providing us with an insider's view of the world of subtitles.

In Part One, Łukasz Bogucki's article outlines familiar approaches to Translation Studies (comparative, process and causal models) and discusses their applicability to AVT research. Special attention is given to a methodology which has already been applied to AVT, namely Action Research. The objective of this paper is to examine whether a universal methodological approach is feasible in the case of a discipline as complex and non-homogeneous as AVT and whether similar tools can be used in studying intra- and interlingual translation, addressing the requirements of diverse audiences.

Lupe Romero discusses issues concerned with the (audiovisual) translation of colloquial speech, with particular reference to cinematographic productions with a high degree of orality (author or independent films). The author proposes a set of categories for analysing colloquial speech and therefore a model, applicable to both dubbing and subtitling, for describing and quantifying the oral features present both in the source and target texts.

Maria Freddi and Silvia Luraghi, followed by Eduard Bartoll, guide us into the world of surtitling: translations or transcriptions projected above the stage or displayed on a screen. Freddi and Luraghi question whether translation universals utilized in subtitling can also be applied to surtitling. With an in-depth analysis of the English translation of Salvatore Cammarano's libretto for Giuseppe Verdi's *Luisa Miller* and a study of translation strategies used therein, the authors propose an interesting avenue of research for universals in translation.

Bartoll's article explores surtitling in an alternative setting – the theatre – and focuses on a Catalan version of *Macbeth*. The author raises awareness of this highly specialized technique and discusses the difficulties of providing surtitles for live performances, which are, of course, subject to changes of rhythm, speed of enunciation and reformulation of dialogue. Bartoll argues that the translator's vulnerability is heightened in this context.

Part Two opens with Claudia Borghetti's contribution, which examines AVT within the framework of Intercultural Foreign Language Education and explores the complex critical-interpretative process that FL students must negotiate in order to translate an AV text. Since this process includes identifying cultural data present in the ST, reflecting on the cultural context of the TT, and deciding if and how to render cultural data on a linguistic level, Borghetti suggests that audiovisual translation can be used effectively in the FL classroom to stimulate students' intercultural awareness.

Continuing along the lines of cultural awareness raised by AVT, Marcella De Marco's contribution offers a different perspective on the utilization of subtitles in academic environments: the author illustrates how gender and identity issues can be integrated in the curriculum design of a subtitling module. The paper presents a subtitling module which constitutes part of the MA in Applied Translation Studies at London Metropolitan University and discusses teaching methodologies and students' reactions.

Moving on to language acquisition *per se*, Eithne O'Connell gives us an overview of the use of AV in language learning and of research into the positive effects that can be derived from this practice. The author then discusses the relevance of such research for minority languages, the Irish language being the case study in question, and how Irish language learners can improve their linguistic skills through the use of subtitled material.

Elisa Perego and Elisa Ghia concentrate on how eye-tracking can be employed to gauge visual attention and reading behaviour of audiences exposed to captions and subtitles. The article reports on experiments showing the impact of different translation strategies and layout format on visual activity and reflects on how results from eye-tracking tests can prove beneficial in FL acquisitional contexts.

Noa Talaván Zanón assesses the benefits of both the creation of interlingual subtitles by the students themselves and the use of ready-made materials. Experiments carried out by the author prove that subtitles are a valid support for enhancing listening comprehension skills in communicative, task-based FL learning contexts.

Expanding on the topic of pedagogical applications of subtitling, Stavroula Sokoli, Patrick Zabalbeascoa and Maria Fountana present the results of an EU-funded project, *Learning via Subtitling*, and discuss the implementation of subtitling activities in third level FL courses. Learners' feedback is analysed and participative learning, through subtitling, is shown to increase students' motivation and attainment.

Finally, after discussions on the validity of using subtitling in FL classes, the closing contribution by Laura Incalcaterra McLoughlin and Jennifer Lertola provides practical guidelines for the implementation of such practice. Whilst examples provided relate to the teaching of Italian, the model can be easily applied to other languages, as the article contains detailed step-by-step descriptions of a typical teaching module unit and required software.

The book concludes with an interview by Carlo Eugeni, an academic and professional subtitler, who gives us an insight into the world of subtitlers and their work. He answers questions on subtitling procedure, standards, "mistakes", and the positive impact of subtitling on translation skills.

Laura Incalcaterra McLoughlin

References

Barthes, R. (1977), *Image-Music-Text*, London: Fontana.
Díaz-Cintas, J. (ed.) (2008), *The Didactics of Audiovisual Translation*. Amsterdam: John Benjamins.
Orero, P. (ed.), *Topics in Audiovisual Translation*. Amsterdam: John Benjamins.

PART ONE

Studies in AVT

ŁUKASZ BOGUCKI

The Application of Action Research to Audiovisual Translation

1. Introduction: Translation research

If one were to draw a mind map to represent translation and notions associated with it, the resulting image would, in all probability, be an aggregate of seemingly unrelated concepts from all walks of life. Computer software, cultural barriers, wordplay, feature films, video games, electronic and traditional dictionaries, ethics, gender, agents of power, termbases, corpora, hermeneutics, neologisms, incompatibility of legal systems – all of these, and many more, have found their way into discussions on translation. Especially recently, with the introduction of new technologies, the meaning of translation has broadened to such an extent that a synonym – localization – is being used more and more frequently (Hatim and Munday, 2004: 113). The non-homogeneity of the concept in question has resulted in a variety of approaches and methodologies that translation researchers have subscribed to.

It is the interdisciplinary nature of translation that has led to a profusion of theoretical approaches, despite the fact that translation studies has only recently been recognized as an academic discipline. From linguistic theories rooted in structuralism and later transformational-generative grammar, through functionalist models, textual approaches, hermeneutics, the cultural turn, psycholinguistics, pragmatics, and gender studies, to cognitive sciences, corpus linguistics and computational linguistics – over the last six or so decades, translation studies has had many faces.

Williams and Chesterman (2002) list three main models of research within translation studies. Comparative models (Catford, 1965; Vinay and

Darbelnet, 1958) are essentially contrastive analyses of source and target languages and / or texts. They tend to be restricted to particular pairs of languages, but have evolved from decontextualized contrastive analyses of small translation units to more detailed and universal studies, like van Leuven-Zwart's approach (1989 and 1990). Process models, which are dynamic as opposed to static comparative models, investigate the relationships between the sender, the translator and the recipient in the process of translation of which Think-Aloud Protocols (Jääskeläinen, 1998) are a typical example. Thirdly, causal models strive to answer the question "why", a key dilemma in translation. The skopos theory or Toury's (1995) normative approach are paragons of this type.

It appears that causal models are the most successful in explaining the complex nature of translation. They help comprehend why translations look the way they do and what it results in (Chesterman, 2000). Chesterman (ibid.: 25) argues further that only a causal model is capable of forming all four kinds of hypotheses necessary in research (viz. interpretive, descriptive, explanatory and predictive); the other two models cannot progress beyond the first two kinds of hypotheses, possibly including predictions in certain cases, but never allowing for explanations.

2. The lure of audiovisual translation

On a side note, it is interesting that major turns in translation studies were more than once preceded by Polish publications, whose reach was limited, but which tackled issues that eventually aroused interest among scholars and instigated changes in approaches or methodologies. Seven years prior to Nida's seminal classic in 1964, Wojtasiewicz published his *Wstęp do teorii tłumaczenia* (Introduction to Translation Theory). This is neither to discredit Nida's achievement nor to go against the popular belief that translation studies indeed started some time around 1964, but it needs to be said that already in 1957 there was a book, albeit in a minority language, that prepared the way for a theory of translation. Similarly, *Les opérations linguistiques qui sous-tendent le processus de sous-titrage des films*, a monograph published in 1993 by Tomaszkiewicz of Poznań is considered to be one of the first books to systematize linguistic issues in the process of subtitling and to open avenues for AVT research.[1] Nine years prior to that, in 1984, when screen translation was virtually *terra incognita*, Hendrykowski published an article on problems in film translation. Again, this is not to say that no mention was made concerning film translation before the 1990s (Dollerup, 1974; Mayoral, 1984); Ivarsson's book appeared one year prior to Tomaszkiewicz's, in 1992; Díaz-Cintas (2004) draws our attention to the existence of an unpublished manuscript on subtitling by Laks dated as early as 1957. However, early publications did not offer any systematic approach to screen translation, often merely listing catalogues of errors in subtitles or at best discussing professional or economic aspects of translating films. Even later publications either concentrated on technical guidelines of subtitling and dubbing as a trade (Dries, 1995) or emphasized the novelty behind these translation types from an academic perspective (Gottlieb, 1997).

Twenty years later, the online bibliography of translation and interpreting managed by the University of Alicante[2] lists 1837 publications devoted to AVT. The number of dissertations on the subject is beyond calculation. Hardly a year passed in the 21st century without at least one international conference on audiovisual translation (Hong Kong 2001, Berlin 2002, London 2004, Barcelona 2005, Copenhagen 2006, Lodz 2007, Leiria 2007, Montpellier 2008, Barcelona 2009, Antwerp 2009, Bologna (Forli) 2010, London 2011, Krakow 2011). However, there are still many unexplored avenues of research, while what has been discussed occasionally suffers from inadequate or superficial treatment. According to Díaz-Cintas (2004: online): "On a research level, the term audiovisual is sometimes added, with

---

1   I am indebted to Henrik Gottlieb for drawing my attention to this book as a precursor to film translation research.

2   BITRA at <https://aplicacionesua.cpd.ua.es/tra_int/usu/buscar.asp?idioma=en> (accessed 19/04/2010).

a certain flippancy to pieces of work to make them more attractive, when in reality what is presented is very limited in its audiovisual specificity and could well be applied to other areas of translation".

It is certainly true that audiovisual translation research is attractive. For a new researcher, it is tempting to list errors in a subtitled movie, illustrating it with screenshots, and even more tempting to suggest improvements. When working on dissertations and term papers pertaining to AVT, bachelor and master students alike may require meticulous guidance so as to go beyond mere error-hunting in a foreign version of another Disney/Pixar production. An experienced supervisor will usually find this fairly easy, but less so when faced with a scarcity of research tools. To quote from Díaz-Cintas's (2004: online) insightful paper again, "many of the translation concepts and theories that have been historically articulated cease to be functional when scholars try and apply them to AVT". One must, however, acknowledge successful attempts at applying translation theories to research in audiovisual translation. The next section will indicate which models of translation have been used to explain screen translation phenomena.

3. Methodologies of AVT research

In his doctoral dissertation, Karamitroglou (2000) posits audiovisual translation (on the example of Greek subtitles) within the framework of norms and polysystem theory. In line with the proponents of translation studies who dismiss the concept of equivalence and prefer instead to discuss norms (cf. the debate in Schäffner, 1999: 32), Karamitroglou discusses the target normative system as being composed of four categories, viz. human agents, products, recipients and audiovisual mode. The application of norms to screen translation appears justified, as professional practice is governed by in-house regulations (e.g. standards observed by film studios in Poland that limit the number of characters in a line of subtitle to between 32 and 40, as well as similar truncations operating in studios across the globe). However, norms in AVT are much more complex than merely technical limitations. Karamitroglou's (2000: 249) conclusion is that audiovisual translation can be researched within the general realm of translation studies.

A similar approach is advocated by Bogucki (2004), who presents a model for analysing cinema subtitles within the framework of Relevance Theory (Sperber and Wilson, 1995). The underlying assumption of the model is that the constraints influencing the subtitler's choice are threefold. Firstly, there are technical constraints. Secondly, there are norms that operate in all forms of translation, as proposed by Toury (1995), for example, and also by Chesterman (1997); and, in this respect, the model is related to that of Karamitroglou. However, thirdly and perhaps most importantly, there is the concept of relevance, which guides the subtitler's actions. The filmic message being typically composed of four semiotic channels (Delabastita, 1989; Gottlieb, 1997) – viz. the picture, music and sound effects, signs and captions and finally the dialogue – its comprehension and appreciation by the audience is a function of the effect that the information conveyed through each of these channels has on the viewers. In plain English, while in certain audiovisual productions one or more of these channels may take precedence over the others (e.g. music being regarded as arguably more important in Kubrick's *2001: A Space Odyssey* than dialogue, the movie being described by the director himself as a "non-verbal experience" (in Castle, 2005)), a film is to be appreciated as a complex whole. Disabled viewers, who are deprived of the possibility of experiencing stimuli coming through some of the channels, can benefit from certain forms of audiovisual translation that make up for this loss (the blind can have the moving picture described to them by means of audio description, as focusing solely on the dialogue, music and sound effects, they would be unable to appreciate the artistic value of the entire semiotic composition). With regard to this peculiarity of audiovisual transfer, choices made by film translators are inevitably filtered by what is relevant, i.e. any redundant elements of film dialogue (information conveyed also by the picture, signs or captions) may well be omitted from the translation. Curtailed by the technical limitations of subtitles and striving for maximum clarity and minimum complexity of message, translators must restrict themselves to what is pertinent. The

Principle of Relevance, arguably applicable to all translation (Gutt, 2000), is thus more applicable to subtitling (Kovačič, 1994).

In her doctoral dissertation, Szarkowska (2007) applied multimodal transcription (Baldry and Thimbault, 2006) to an analysis of Polish soap operas subtitled into English. Multimodality surpasses language to demonstrate that communication is also possible through sound, music, image and gestures. An application of multimodal analysis to audiovisual translation seems methodologically appropriate in the light of the semiotic composition of film discussed above. The visual frames of the audiovisual material are juxtaposed with a meticulous description of each, including time frame, information on camera position, perspective, visual focus, distance, visually salient items, colours, coding orientation as well as kinesic action of participants, soundtrack and a metafunctional interpretation of meaning. This approach was first placed in the audiovisual context by Taylor (2004).

Research into audiovisual translation poses a challenge in that the domain under scrutiny is semiotically and technically complex. Translation *per se* is an interdisciplinary activity, while film translation carries the added factor of merging the visual with the verbal. As Munday (2001: 189) notes, "the construction of an interdisciplinary methodology is not straightforward, since few researchers possess the necessary expertise in a wide range of subject areas". Furthermore, though all kinds of translations are done with the target recipient in mind and quality assessment models often take into account what the audience make of the foreign language versions (House in Baker and Saldanha, 2009: 222), it seems that in screen translation the audience's opinion should be of prime importance. Many surveys such as Inst. SMG KRC Poland (Bogucki, 2004: 12), European Barometer (Gambier, 2006) or TGI Latina[3] indicate viewers' preferences as regards particular types of audiovisual transfer. It seems necessary, therefore, to consider a methodology that is versatile, flexible and recipient-centred. Action Research seems a good candidate.

---

3   <http://www.zonalatina.com/Zldata163.htm> (accessed 01/10/2010).

4. Action Research

Action Research (AR) is a multifaceted concept. It is regarded by many theorists (Coghlan and Brannick, 2001) as a generic term for a number of forms of research geared at action. The two nouns that make up the name indicate that this methodology (or indeed collection of methodologies) concentrates on acting (and thus changing the present state of affairs) and researching (and thus understanding the problems involved).

The concept of action has already been utilized in translation studies, notably by Holz-Mänttäri (1984), whose model of translatorial action was based on action theory, an approach not unrelated to Action Research (for a discussion of action theory and AR, see Mayhew, 1968). The two main characteristics of AR are that it is participative and cyclic (Cravo and Neves, 2007). Firstly, it involves active participation on the part of members of the system under scrutiny (Wadsworth, 1998); secondly, problem-solving is not linear, but repetitive.

As far as translation studies are concerned, AR is essentially an attempt to bridge the gap between theory and practice. When applied to translational research, the methodology would not concern abstract issues like equivalence, but practical problems affecting translators. In Hatim's (2001: 7) words, "translation studies is seeking to promote the stance that research is not only something to be done to or on practitioners, but is also something done by practitioners". This is a very valid point, as the routes of theoreticians and practitioners exploring the nature of translation tend to fork only too often, or indeed, run parallel from the very start. It seems that in AVT in particular, combining the expertise of practising translators with the broad knowledge of translation theoreticians would be fruitful.

One characteristic of AR that renders it particularly suitable for audiovisual translation is its cyclic nature combined with reflections upon each ensuing cycle of research. Action Research seems to be an ongoing process, as while trying to solve a particular problem, the researcher frequently encounters new ones. This spiral of revisions and constant development appears necessary in an area as dynamic and varied as AVT. Technological

development brings about new, previously unimaginable types of audiovisual transfer such as live subtitling. The internet has dramatically influenced
amateur subtitling known as fansubbing. Cinema subtitles are no longer
chemically produced. Audience preferences are changing over longer periods of time; voice-over as we know it may eventually disappear from Polish
television (Bogucki, 2010). Specialized software greatly facilitates alterations
to the font, colour and positioning of subtitles. Sophisticated computer
graphics make it possible to render animated characters so realistically that
lip-synchronization in dubbing becomes an issue.

Possible shortcomings of AR include its limited relevance. Cohen
and Manion (1980: 216) point out that the findings of AR are usually
applicable only to a specific situation. Thus far, applications of AR to the
area of audiovisual transfer have largely concentrated on particular sub-
types rather than on the entire subdiscipline. Szarkowska (forthcoming)
discusses the use of AR in subtitling for the deaf and hard-of-hearing. She
describes how research involving three groups – the hearing-impaired,
AVT professionals and researchers – can lead to improving the quality of
intralingual subtitles.

5. AR in teaching audiovisual translation

The gap between theory and practice is not only seen in translation itself,
but also in translator training. While many institutions do realize the
practical potential of translation, offering hands-on training for future
and beginner translators taught by experienced practitioners with the
help of sophisticated tools, others focus on theoretical aspects, often limiting the practice to getting students to translate texts and marking their
assignments. The problem may largely be due to the fact that translation
is often part of language studies curricula. On occasions, philology graduates teach translation classes without clear guidelines as to whether they
are supposed to merely help their students improve language skills through

translation-related activities or whether their role is to train translators. However, to a certain extent, it is a financial issue since translators are reluctant to lend their expertise to higher education institutions as they make more money translating than teaching. Moreover, the cost of translation software and modern computer equipment may inhibit universities in poorer countries.

Although some European universities are beginning to offer degrees in AVT, in this respect the map of Europe is largely filled with blank spots. Despite the interest in audiovisual translation in Poland, teaching AVT is in its infancy, if not only in its conceptual phase. The two main characteristics of Action Research, active participation and cyclic nature, make it a potential candidate for inclusion in syllabi. Institutions contemplating the inception of AVT courses and degrees should probably consider this approach. A similar view is expressed by Cravo and Neves (2007).

6. Conclusions

A uniform methodological approach to audiovisual translation does not appear feasible. There may be certain similarities between the three main modes of audiovisual transfer, but even within that paradigm the differences are more striking, for example the change in mode from speech to writing in the case of subtitling, the additive nature of this type of translation, the applicable constraints and target audience preferences regarding the use of subtitles, dubbing and voice-over. The less common kinds of AVT cater for limited audiences and are technically quite diverse. There may be intralingual aids for disabled viewers, like audio description and subtitling for the deaf and hard-of-hearing (SDH); their scope may be heavily restricted in terms of both audience and content type, like surtitling; like live subtitling, they may rely on advanced technology and skills beyond the realm of translation competence. Technological advances may eventually render AVT even less homogeneous than it is today. Having said that, research within AVT should probably be based on causal models involving the audience. The versatility of AR makes it a viable platform to guide research into audiovisual translation, as well as practical courses within this area.

References

Baldry, A. and P. Thimbault (2006), *Multimodal Transcription and Text Analysis. A Multimedia Toolkit and Coursebook with Associated On-line Course*. London: Equinox.

Bogucki, Ł. (2004), *A Relevance Framework for Constraints on Cinema Subtitling*. Łódź: Łódź University Press.

—— (2010), The Demise of Voice-over? Audiovisual Translation in Poland in the 21st Century. In B. Lewandowska-Tomaszczyk and M. Thelen (eds), *Meaning in Translation*, Lodz Studies in Language vol. 19. Frankfurt am Main: Peter Lang.

Castle A. (2005), *The Stanley Kubrick Archives*. Köln: Taschen.

Catford, J. C. (1965), *A Linguistic Theory of Translation: An Essay in Applied Linguistics*. Oxford: Oxford University Press.

Chesterman, A. (1997), *Memes of Translation. The Spread of Ideas in Translation Theory*. Amsterdam: John Benjamins.

—— (2000) A Causal Model for Translation Studies. In M. Olohan (ed.) (2000), *Intercultural Faultiness – Research Models in Translation Studies I – Textual and Cognitive Aspects*. Manchester: St Jerome, 15–26.

Coghlan, D. and T. Brannick (2001), *Doing Action Research in your Own Organization*. London: Sage Publications.

Cohen, L. and L. Manion (1980), *Research Methods in Education*. London: Croom Helm.

Cravo, A. and J. Neves (2007), Action Research in Translation Studies. *The Journal of Specialised Translation* 7, 92–107.

Delabastita, D. (1989), Translation and Mass-Communication: Film and TV Translation as Evidence of Cultural Dynamics. *Babel* 35(4), 193–218.

Díaz-Cintas, J. (2004), Subtitling: the Long Journey to Academic Acknowledgement. *The Journal of Specialised Translation* 1, 50–70.

Dollerup, C. (1974), On Subtitles in Television Programmes. *Babel* 20, 197–202.

Dries, J. (1995), *Dubbing and Subtitling: Guidelines for Production and Distribution*. Düsseldorf: European Institute for the Media.

Gambier, Y. (2006), Multimodality and Audiovisual Translation. *MuTra* 2006: Audiovisual Translation Scenarios, conference proceedings, <http://www.euroconferences.info/proceedings/2006_Proceedings/2006_Gambier_Yves.pdf>.

Gottlieb, H. (1997), *Subtitles, Translation & Idioms*. Copenhagen: University of Copenhagen.

Gutt, E. A. (2000), *Translation and Relevance: Cognition and Context*. Manchester: St. Jerome Publishing.

Hatim, B. (2001), *Teaching and Researching Translation*. Harlow: Pearson Education Limited.

Hatim, B. and J. Munday (2004), *Translation. An Advanced Resource Book*. London: Routledge.

Hendrykowski, M. (1984) Z problemów przekładu filmowego. In E. Balcerzan (ed.), *Wielojęzyczność Literatury a Problemy Przekładu Artystycznego*. Wrocław: Ossolineum, 243–59.

Ivarsson, J. (1992), *Subtitling for the Media*. Simrisham: TransEdit.

Jääskeläinen, R. (1998), Think-aloud Protocol. In M. Baker and K. Malmkjaer (eds), *Routledge Encyclopedia of Translation Studies*. London: Routledge, 265–9.

Karamitroglou, F. (2000) *Towards a Methodology for the Investigation of Norms in Audiovisual Translation*. Amsterdam: Rodopi.

Kovačič, I. (1994), Relevance as a Factor in Subtitling Reductions. In C. Dollerup and A. Lindegaard (eds), *Teaching Translation and Interpreting 2*. Amsterdam: John Benjamins, 245–52.

Leuven-Zwart, K. van (1989), Translation and Original: Similarities and Dissimilarities, I. *Target 1: 2*, 151–81.

—— (1990), Translation and Original: Similarities and Dissimilarities, II. *Target 2: 1*, 69–95.

Mayhew, L. (1968), Action Theory and Action Research. *Social Problems* 15(4), 420–32.

Mayoral, A. R. (1984), La traducción y el cine. El subtítulo. *Babel: revista de los estudiantes de la EUTI 2*, 16–26.

Munday, J. (2001), *Introducing Translation Studies. Theories and Applications*. London: Routledge.

Nida, E. (1964), *Toward a Science of Translating*. Leiden: Brill.

Schäffner, Ch. (ed.) (1999), *Translation and Norms*. Clevedon: Multilingual Matters.

Sperber, D. and D. Wilson (1995), *Relevance: Communication and Cognition* (2nd edn). Oxford: Blackwell.

Szarkowska, A. (2007), *Forms of Address in Contemporary English and Polish: Implications for Translation*. Unpublished doctoral dissertation, University of Warsaw.

—— (2009), Nowe podejścia metodologiczne w przekładzie audiowizualnym. In K. Hejwowski, A. Szczęsny and U. Topczewska (eds), 50 lat poskiej translatoryki. Warszawa: ILS, 591–602.

Taylor, Ch. (2004), Multimodal Text Analysis and Subtitling. In E. Ventola, C. Charles and M. Kaltenbacher (eds), *Perspectives on Multimodality*. Amsterdam: John Benjamins, 153–72.

Tomaszkiewicz, T. (1993), *Les opérations linguistiques qui sous-tendent le processus de sous-titrage des films*. Poznań: Wydawnictwo UAM.

Toury, G. (1995), *Descriptive Translation Studies and Beyond*. Amsterdam: John Benjamins.

Vinay, J.-P., and J. Darbelnet (1995[1958]), *Stylistique comparée du français et de l'anglais. Méthode de traduction*. Paris: Didier, trans. and ed. J. C. Sager and M.-J. Hamel (1995) as *Comparative Stylistics of French and English: A Methodology for Translation*. Amsterdam: John Benjamins.

Wadsworth, Y. (1998), What is Participatory Action Research? *Action Research International*, Paper 2.

Williams, J., and A. Chesterman (2002), *The Map: A Beginner's Guide to Doing Research in Translation Studies*. Manchester: St Jerome Publishing.

Wojtasiewicz, O. (1996[1957]), *Wstęp do teorii tłumaczenia*. Warszawa: TEPIS.

LUPE ROMERO

When Orality Is Less Pre-fabricated: An Analytical Model for the Study of Colloquial Conversation in Audiovisual Translation

1. Introduction

The translation of colloquial speech is raising constant interest in the field of audiovisual translation, with special attention accorded to the translation of those fictional genres in which the characters' language is strongly characterized by the use of everyday colloquial expressions. However, it is widely known that the creation of such dialogues, both in the source text and in the target text, is based on a previous script. Several authors (Chaume, 2001 and 2004; Mason, 1989; Whitman-Linsen, 1992) have stressed that audiovisual translation creates realistic, natural and acceptable dialogues by including certain oral features and by explicitly excluding others which, although pertaining to authentic spontaneous speech, cannot be included in a prepared or "pre-fabricated" discourse (Chaume, 2004: 168) for their written nature. However, in some cinematographic productions, which are known as "author films" or "independent films", directors decide to use a language marked by a certain degree of orality with aesthetic, realistic, expressive or ideological purposes. In several of these films, the director is also the scriptwriter and, sometimes, the main character. Therefore, even if dialogues are based on a written script, they are constantly evolving during filming. This consideration leads us to claim that oral features may not respond to the necessity of representing a "real" colloquial conversation but they could be used for other purposes.

The aim of this paper is to propose a series of categories for analysing informal, colloquial speech in cinematographic productions in which the purpose of oral features is not limited to the representation of spontaneous discourse. The model we propose includes all oral features at every language level and it has been designed from a translational perspective, with the purpose of describing and quantifying oral features present in the ST and in the TT analysed. Moreover, these categories allow analysis of both spoken and written text phenomena and can be used for the analysis of colloquial speech in dubbing as well as in subtitling.

2. Spontaneous colloquial speech versus pre-fabricated orality

Most of the research carried out in AVT in Spain is based on Chaume's model (2004) and on the concept of "pre-fabricated orality", whose main assumption is that the oral features present in source and target text dialogues pertain, in fact, to a written register which endeavours to sound as if it were oral. Due to its nature, which has been described as "written to be spoken as if not written" (Gregory and Carroll, 1978: 42) or "planned to be written and to eventually be acted as if not written" (Romero Fresco, 2008), "pre-fabricated" discourse differs from spontaneous speech in that it presents a limited number of colloquial features, which contribute to spontaneous-sounding conversation. In the case of AVT, source language dialogues must be plausible and the translator must reflect spontaneous speech in the target language as well as adhering to the conventions of the translation mode being used.

Most of these conventions are listed in a style guide called *Criteris lingüístics sobre traducció i doblatge* (Linguistic criteria for translation and dubbing) published in 1997 by the Catalan channel Televisió de Catalunya (TVC). Although this guide only refers to the Catalan language, Chaume (2004) points out that it can also be applied to Spanish dubbing. This style guide recommends that translators use a register which is colloquial but "controlled" by applying linguistic techniques such as coordination and juxtaposition, as well as interruptions, topicalizations, ellipsis, deixis and stereotypical structures which correspond to specific communicative situations, among others. Moreover, translators are advised to avoid other colloquial features typical of spontaneous speech, such as redundancies and digressions (TVC, 1997: 12, 14). Chaume (2004: 168) generally supports the guidelines proposed by TVC and remarks that these recommendations may also be applied to subtitling, although they have been designed for dubbing. Following Chaume, other researchers (Matamala, 2004; Baños, 2006; Cuenca, 2008; Romero Fresco, 2008) have studied the differences between pre-fabricated oral discourse in original cinema productions and pre-fabricated oral discourse in Spanish and/or Catalan dubbing, as well as specific features of orality, such as the translation of interjections, discourse markers etc.

These studies are correct in claiming that, if the colloquial features of the source dialogues are pre-fabricated and respond to the conventions of cinema and the linguistic conventions of the SL, then, it is logical to expect that the translation of these dialogues follows the same conventions in the TL. But, what happens if the source text does not follow this rule, that is, if SL dialogues are deliberately spontaneous and informal? In this case, we are likely to find several features of colloquial oral discourse, such as redundancies, repetitions or digressions which, according to Chaume, are generally not found in pre-fabricated texts. What about translation? Should professionals translate these dialogue exchanges as if they were pre-fabricated or should they reflect the author's intention and find equivalent solutions? In this paper, we endeavour to answer these questions by proposing a model for analysing different categories of informal colloquial speech. This model will help us discover whether these colloquial features were deliberately used by the original author and whether the translated texts have reflected the purpose of the source text by using equivalent colloquial solutions.

3. Methodology and corpus

The categories we propose for analysing informal, colloquial speech are based on empirical research (Romero, 2010), which combines qualitative and quantitative data to describe linguistic variety.[1] One of the main objectives of this study is to investigate how translators deal with linguistic variety problems in dubbing and subtitling from Italian into Spanish. The corpus used is characterized by linguistic variety features with a specific aim and the categories of analysis used allow us to describe and quantify both the characteristics of the ST and solutions used in the TT.

The corpus analysed is the film *Il postino* (*The Postman*), both in its original Italian version and in its translations into Spanish, one of which is dubbed and three are subtitled. *Il postino* was chosen as the corpus for this study because it fulfils four fundamental requirements.

First of all, the film was written and starred by one of the major representatives of Italian comedy, Massimo Troisi, whose works are characterized by a remarkable use of language, which includes features of Neapolitan dialect and of the oral and popular register, a factor that helps create a spontaneous oral discourse and an informal tone.

Secondly, Troisi uses colloquial speech and dialect for different purposes, which sometimes overlap. Based on the considerations of various authors (Coluccia, 1996; Verardi, 1996; Sommario, 2004), we concluded that Troisi uses both informal colloquial speech and dialect for the following purposes: creating authentic conversation by reproducing spontaneous speech with which the spectator can identify; innovating through utilizing natural and spontaneous language which differs from the language used in

---

1   This model of categories for analysing colloquial speech is based on Romero's PhD thesis (2010), which develops an empirical study of the translation of linguistic variety in dubbing and subtitling. The analysis includes the study of the source text and the target text in relation to the presence of geographic and social dialect, as well as informal colloquial speech. It also develops a quantitative and qualitative analysis of the formal constraints of subtitling, in order to establish whether the formal presentation of subtitles influences linguistic variety.

most of the films based on a script; creating a specific socio-cultural profile for his characters, who are usually moderately educated persons and are not linguistically trained, making it difficult for them to talk concisely (Romero, 2010).

Thirdly, Troisi's dialogues usually evolve. Pavignano, the scriptwriter for most of Troisi's films, points out that written dialogues were merely used as a guide since during the actual shooting, Troisi used his own words to express these ideas (in Sommario 2004: 187). Improvisation and lack of "pre-fabrication" in Troisi's dialogues are also noted by Ratford, the director of *Il postino* (*Il postino*, subtitle 41, director's comment on the first scene).

Fourthly, the film gained international recognition and this allowed us to collect data on the factors that influenced its translation, such as distribution, reception and the importance attributed to language. This final factor was determinant, since *Il postino*, unlike other films written by Troisi, was distributed in Spain both in its dubbed and subtitled version.

In order to obtain data on the reasons why the director decided to use colloquial and dialectic features, we decided to carry out a linguistic analysis of the dialogues of Mario, the protagonist of the film (interpreted by Troisi himself) and who presents the highest number of exchanges (218). His dialogues are also rich in colloquial and dialectal expressions.

The analysis we propose has been preceded by a pilot study based on an analytical model created by Briz (1998) to study Spanish colloquial speech. The objective of this study was to establish relevant categories for the analysis of the whole corpus. The categories we isolated were selected from a translational perspective and allowed us to obtain qualitative and quantitative data on the reasons for using informal colloquial features in the ST, on the linguistic differences between the original and the translated versions, on the influence of the translation mode (dubbing and subtitling), on the presence of linguistic variety features and, finally, on the categories of informal speech used in each translated version. This article aims to present a model for the analysis of informal colloquial speech.

4. Spanish colloquial conversation: Briz's model (1998)

The categories proposed in this paper for the analysis of informal colloquial speech in translation are based on Briz's pragmatic model (1998), which analyses Spanish colloquial conversation (see Table 1). This model was chosen for different reasons:

- The object of this study. Briz sees colloquial Spanish as a modality of speech characterized by a spontaneous oral mode, an informal tone, common everyday topics and an interactive tenor. This definition is suitable for our study, since Troisi's language presents similar characteristics.
- The categories. Briz establishes concrete categories whose purpose is to systematize and create a pragmatic "grammar" of colloquial speech. These categories, grouped in strategies, are operational units for our analysis, which is based on the identification of informal colloquial markers in the ST and on the identification of corresponding solutions in the TT.
- Contrastivity. The strategies determined by Briz to describe colloquial Spanish include features identified by Italian authors to describe Italian oral speech. Therefore, Briz's model is very useful in order to carry out a contrastive analysis, since oral features can be identified and described both in the Italian and in the Spanish versions, using the same categories. Table 1 illustrates the categories including linguistic phenomena identified by Berruto (1985), Sabatini (1985), Berretta (1994) and Bazzanella (1994). These phenomena do not include spoken Italian features that are uncharacteristic of colloquial register (such as the pronouns *lui, lei* etc. used instead of *egli, ella,* since the latter are used only in formal written texts), nor those linguistic phenomena pertaining to the user's social level (such as the use of erroneous structures caused by the interference of similar constructions) since most of these cases are related to socio-cultural factors.

Table 1: Correspondences between strategies in informal colloquial Spanish and the general characteristics of spoken Italian

Briz's model of colloquial Spanish (1998)	Characteristics of spoken Italian adapted from Berruto (1985), Sabatini (1985), Berretta (1994) and Bazzanella (1994)
Syntactic or construction strategies: concatenated syntax, fragmentation, explicative paraphrases, open syntactic links, redundancy, direct style and pragmatic order.	Extensive use of juxtaposition and coordination instead of subordination.
	Paraphrases and repetitions.
	Constructions with *c'è/ci sono + che.*
	Pronominal redundancy (*ci + avere;*).
	Polyvalent use of *che.*
	Fragmented discourse.
	Syntactic emphasis: *dislocazione a destra e a sinistra* (anticipation and postposition) and *la frase scissa* (truncated).
Contextual strategies: ellipsis, deixis and interruption.	Ellipsis and deixis.
	Anacoluthon.
Tense and mode strategies: change in verbal tense and mode.	Preferences in the use of verbal tenses and modes (relative clause or gerund instead of present participle; absence of passive forms).
	Preferences in the use of verbal tenses (present, imperfect with different values, *passato prossimo* to express past actions and rare use of the future tense).
	Preferences in the use of certain verbal tenses (imperfect, present and future).
Phonetic strategies: intonation, pauses, phonetic elongation, marked and emphatic pronunciation, phonetic hesitations.	Filled pauses (phonetic elongation and expressions such as *hmm, ehm*).
	Empty pauses (silences).

Lexical-semantic strategies and constants: lexical frequency and argot.	Generic lexicon.
	Verbal periphrases with time and modal verbs to express future actions.
Production and reception strategies: linguistic intensification and attenuation.	Adjectives and deictic features used as a means of intensification.
	Attenuating or intensifying expressions.
	Approximate or generalizing expressions.
	Impersonal and generic constructions (use of the passive form with no agent or impersonal *si*).
Connection, argumentation and formulation strategies: argumentative or metadiscursive pragmatic connectors.	Discourse markers: particles, interjections, mechanisms for opening or closing sentences, fillers etc.
	Markers with an interactive or metadiscursive function (turn exchange, attention, phatic function, agreement, demarcation, emphasis, and reformulation).

5. Problems encountered in the pilot study

Once we had established that Briz's analytic model was suitable for our study, we undertook a pilot study in which we analysed 65 dialogue exchanges (out of 218 which constituted the whole corpus) by using the categories proposed by the author. This was done to verify that such categories could be applied to a textual analysis from a translation studies perspective.

The problems we encountered were mainly due to the fact that our specific requirements differed from Briz's study. Our analysis, in fact, aims at establishing categories which are suitable for a translational analysis, linguistic categories which are both discrete and mutually exclusive and which serve to identify colloquial features in the ST and compare them to solutions applied by translators in the TT. In this sense, the pragmatic nature of Briz's model constituted an obstacle to this objective. The specific problems encountered were:

Firstly, although Briz establishes linguistic categories, they have a fundamentally pragmatic nature. The model has a pragmatic approach which is primarily based on the concepts of function and user's intention; therefore, one linguistic category may correspond to different pragmatic categories. For example, syllable elongation is a phonetic strategy; however, if it is used to stress the meaning (pragmatic criterion), it may be regarded as an intensification strategy. At the same time, one pragmatic category may include various linguistic categories. For example, in Briz's model, lexical frequency, which pertains to lexical-semantic strategies, includes lexical units with extended meaning, which systematically replace more specific units, as well as socially or metaphorically marked units. Therefore, the same "label" may include various linguistic categories, such as discourse markers (*primero* instead of *en primer lugar*); lexical units (*sitio* instead of *lugar*), morphosyntactic structures (*tener ganas* instead of *desear*) and intensifying lexemes (*horrible, montón, cantidad*), utilized in order to emphasize or criticize other people's actions (pragmatic criterion).

The analysis of translation could be based on function or on user's purpose; however, the fact that one function may include different categories or, vice versa, that one category may respond to different functions, constitutes an obstacle to a contrastive analysis of the colloquial features identified in the ST and in the TT.

Briz's categories are not discrete or mutually exclusive. In fact, some of them overlap because descriptions and definitions are identical. As an example, we can mention concatenated syntax, fragmentation, explicative paraphrases and open syntactic links, which are syntactic or construction strategies. Briz (1998: 68, my translation)[2] defines concatenated syntax as an "accumulation of utterances" resulting from a lack of planning, while fragmentation is described as a "concatenation and accumulation of utterances"

---

2   All translations are mine unless otherwise indicated.

(ibid.: 69) due to the user's need to explain something exhaustively in order
to ensure its correct interpretation. Explicative paraphrases are defined as a
"slow progress of information [through] paraphrases, concatenated or accu-
mulated details, extremely accurate descriptions, parenthetical insertions,
judgments, etc." (ibid.: 70–1) and they are also linked to the user's desire to
explain something in detail and ensure correct understanding. Finally, an
open syntactic link is described as a "weak bond between utterances", which
allows the speaker to "make repetitions, add commentaries and reiterate,
expand, explain and justify certain arguments", etc. (ibid.: 75).

As we can see, these four categories overlap because all of them are
characterized by the definition "accumulation of utterances" and they are
not differentiated by any features. From a pragmatic perspective, they all
derive from the user's need to explain, expand, justify etc. However, from
a linguistic perspective, Briz does not clarify which textual or syntactic
mechanisms lead to this accumulation of utterances.

Our study needs discrete and mutually exclusive categories, that is,
categories which are clearly defined and diverse and allow identifying colloquial features both in the ST and in the TT. Following the pilot study
undertaken using Briz's model, we established a set of categories which
were suitable for an analysis of translation and which assisted in analysing
colloquial features in conversation. Their general characteristics are:

(1) The term "strategy", used by Briz to define the groups of categories,
     was suppressed, since it refers to function and user's purpose and
     responds to the author's pragmatic approach in the definition of col-
     loquial speech linguistic phenomena. In translation studies, however,
     "strategy" refers to the mechanisms used to solve problems during
     the translation process and, therefore, it is not a suitable term from a
     translational perspective.

(2) Secondly, we abandoned his fundamentally pragmatic definition of
     categories. As mentioned above, a pragmatic approach does not allow
     for describing phenomena based on purely linguistic features, since
     such phenomena are classified by the user's intention. Our classifica-
     tion, instead, includes categories which describe and define specific

linguistic phenomena and do not consider the speaker's intention, allowing for a more suitable translational analysis.

(3) Finally, we suppressed overlapping categories. Our pilot study demonstrated that some of the categories proposed by Briz overlapped because definitions were based on the speaker's intention. Speech can respond to different purposes, depending on whether the speaker wishes to justify, evaluate, emphasize or minimize something and these purposes can lead to different linguistic phenomena. For example, Briz considers that both anticipated information and repeated utterances respond to the speakers' willingness to emphasize what they are going to say or what they have just said, respectively. From a pragmatic point of view, the definition of these categories is identical, since the speaker's intention is similar in both cases. However, from a linguistic perspective, they can be perfectly separated and one linguistic phenomenon can be used for different purposes. For instance, Briz considers that an interruption can be either described as an intensifying feature to strengthen the utterance or the user's attitude or as a means of minimizing the speaker's responsibility. However, from a linguistic perspective, an interruption does not depend on the speaker's intention. Our proposal, based on linguistic criteria to define and characterize colloquial features, avoids the overlapping of categories and helps identify and compare colloquial speech in the ST and in translation.

6. An analytical model for the study of colloquial conversation in AVT

Our model is based on a general characterization of colloquial speech containing redundancies, repetitions and accumulation of utterances, paraphrasing, amplifications, explications, justifications, reformulations etc. These general features have a linguistic correspondent in specific colloquial features which are grouped in discrete and mutually exclusive categories.

This means that each linguistic unit analysed can only pertain to one category. For example, amplification of information is a textual feature which is achieved through a specific colloquial feature, such as cohesion with juxtaposition (only if utterances appear between commas), cohesion with discourse markers (only if utterances are linked by discourse markers) or cohesion with repetition (only if the second utterance is a repetition of the first one or if it refers to the first one). Obviously, the same linguistic unit can assume a different role depending on context. The Spanish *mira* or *ahora* have a referential meaning, since they represent the imperative form of the verb *mirar* and a time adverb, respectively; however, in a specific context, they can act as discourse markers. We can also find utterances or features with two colloquial features, as in the case of *buenoo*, a discourse marker characterized, in turn, by phonetic elongation. Therefore, when we claim that our categories are mutually exclusive, we do not suggest that a linguistic unit can have only one colloquial feature, but that these categories do not overlap and are clearly distinguished, since each of them corresponds to a specific phenomenon whose linguistic definition in a specific context is unique.

Our proposal includes five groups of categories of colloquial features: (1) textual organization features, (2) morphosyntactic features; (3) lexical features; (4) paralinguistic features; (5) phonetic features (only for the oral mode: the analysis of the ST and the dubbed version); (6) graphic features denoting orality (only for the written mode: the analysis of subtitled versions).

6.1. Textual organization features

These features serve as referents or connectors and give cohesion to utterances. An utterance is defined as the formulation of an idea with a full and complete meaning, regardless of whether it is a noun phrase or a verb phrase (that is, with or without a verb). Textual organization features are divided into eight categories:

6.1.1. Cohesion with juxtaposition. Utterances are linked through juxtaposition, regardless of their function (paraphrasing, amplifying, explicating, justifying etc.). In this case, cohesion between utterances is not due to the presence of connectors.

Examples:[3]

R.194	VO: Tanto qua, pure quando hai spezzato le catene, ma *dove vai, che fai?*
	VD: Sí, pero aquí cuando has roto tus cadenas, *¿adónde vas, qué haces?*

6.1.2. Cohesion with discourse markers. These utterances are linked by discourse markers. They can be oral connectors (which, unlike written markers, are redundant or introduce redundant utterances) or elements whose meaning is not referential and is fixed by the context of conversation (*eh; ya; luego*): the latter also act as oral connectors. Discourse markers are not fixed, since they can be placed at the beginning, in the middle or at the end of a sentence and the type of marker used varies depending on their function: arguing, explaining, rejecting, amplifying etc.

Examples:

R.34	VO: *Cioè*, Voi dite che non la può cancellare e riscriverla meglio.
	VOSEA: *O sea,/¿*Vd. dice que no puede borrarla/y escribir otra.

6.1.3. Intensification of discourse markers. These features act as emphasizers in utterances which are linked by discourse markers and stress their meaning.

---

3   These examples are taken from the corpus analysed and they correspond to Mario's exchanges. The examples taken from the subtitled versions are formed by more than one subtitle and the feature analysed is in Italic type in each example. Abbreviations mean: R (character's exchange number); VO (Italian original version); VD (dubbed version in Spanish); VOSEA (subtitled Spanish version for the cinema); VOSEB (subtitled Spanish version for DVD); VOSEC (subtitled Spanish version distributed in Brazil on DVD). Finally, a single slash (/) separates the first and the second line in a subtitle of two lines.

Examples:

R.75	VO: *E allora*, allora è, allora è troppo. VOSEB: *Entonces es que/* necesita demasiada.

6.1.4. Cohesion with repetition. These utterances are repetitive or redundant and are not linked by connectors: the second utterance has a referential relation to the first one.

Examples:

R.1	VO: Però loro dicono che questo qua *è un paese ricco, un paese* che si lavora, *un paese ...* VOSEC: Pero dicen que/*es un país rico donde* hay trabajo, *un país--*

6.1.5. Deixis. These features refer to the immediate environment of speech. The speaker uses these features to signal or indicate different discourse elements in an immediate, contemporary or previous context (place adverbs: *aquí, allí, qua, là etc.*; modal adverbs: *así, cosi etc.*; personal pronouns: *yo, nosotros, io, noi etc.*; demonstrative pronouns: *este, aquel etc.*). These features refer to immediate, contemporary or very recent scenes in the film and they can be replaced by the noun they refer to or understood by the context. Therefore their use is redundant. This analysis deliberately does not take into account deictic features related to a normative, non-redundant use, that is, features which refer to elements introducing new information and which cannot be understood by the context (*ayer, mañana, ieri, domani etc.*). Although they are deictic features, they are not necessarily colloquial.

Examples:

R.177	VO: A che è venuto *qua, quello?* VOSEB: ¿A qué ha venido *ése?*

6.1.6. Ellipsis. This textual cohesion procedure is defined by the absence of certain elements in the textual chain. The elided feature may be an utterance, a noun or a verb, although the first case is the most frequent in colloquial speech. In the following example, the elided part is presented in square brackets:

Examples:

R.17	VO: Buon giorno. [*Le porto la*] Posta. VOSEA: Buenos días. [*Le traigo el*] Correo.

6.1.7. Direct speech. Direct discourse utterances in speech. An excessive presence of this feature is an indicator of the presence of social dialect, since the speakers' socio-cultural level prevents them from using indirect speech.

Examples:

R.23	VO: *"Amor"*, pure se, per esempio, sta lontano così si chiamano proprio: *"amor, amor"*. VOSEC: *"Amor"*. Aunque estén lejos se llaman *"amor"*/el uno al otro.

6.1.8. Cohesion with pauses. They are produced when the speaker remains silent for some time before answering a question, an order, a request etc. or when there is a pause between utterances and the pause acts as a cohesive element (which is not the case in predictable syntactic pauses). These pauses can be identified as a cohesive feature either because the preceding utterance is incomplete or because the following utterance is redundant. Cohesive pauses may be placed before or after a discourse marker or they may even replace it. This category has been included in our classification, as it has been observed that, in some cases, pauses are not a mere phonetic phenomenon but have a clear cohesive value. However, this category has not been included in our analysis, since the distinction between both types of pauses was not always clear and, therefore, data would not have been "clean". In fact, the difference between cohesive and phonetic pauses merits deeper study.[4] In this example, pauses are indicated by two slashes:

Examples:

R.188	VO: Vai // continua, va' VD: Sigue // Continúa. VOSEA: Vamos, sigue, *hombre*.

6.2. Morphosyntactic features

These colloquial features modify speech at a morphological or syntactical level. These features include seven categories:

6.2.1. Interruption. This category includes anacoluthon which is a change in syntax, and the interruption of utterances with a complete illocutive value. This category also includes involuntary interruptions caused by the speaker.

Examples:

R.1	VO: Ho un raffreddore stamattina e … Avrò preso umidità, no? sulla barca quando so' salito. *Come metto i piedi su quella barca io* … (…) Come fai tu a stare notte e giorno sopra e non pigli mai niente. *Io, come ci salgo* … VOSEA: Desde por la mañana/tengo catarro. Habré cogido humedad/en la barca, no lo sé. Mire, *en cuanto pongo pie/en esa barca, yo* … ¿Cómo puedes tú pasarte día y noche/encima de esa …? Y nunca coges nada. *Yo en cuanto subo* …

---

4   The analysis of silences has traditionally been a psychological domain, although it has recently attracted the interest of psycholinguistics and conversation analysis (Maclay and Osgood, 1959; Sacks et al., 1974; Butterworth, 1980; Poyatos, 1980; Quilis and Hernández Alonso, 1990; Valle Arroyo, 1991). These authors have carried out various analyses and classifications of the concept of silence in conversation. Due to the complexity of the object of study and the necessity of further instruments of analysis, our research on pauses has been confined to the identification of non-syntactical pauses, without specifying whether they only have a phonetic or a cohesive value.

6.2.2. Marked order. This category includes utterances characterized by an unconventional word order, with items placed before or after their usual position or with syntactic structures which emphasize certain features by placing them before their usual position.

Examples:

R.193	VO: *La guerra*, la vinciamo noi.
	VD: *La guerra*, la ganaremos nosotros.

6.2.3. Morphosyntactic intensification. These features are emphatic or redundant morphological units or informal constructions. This category includes features of intensification which are typical of oral speech, but also features which can be found in written texts (indirect pronouns, augmentative suffixes, adverbs, reflexive forms of transitive verbs etc.) These features are quantified in our study when they are redundant (characteristic of colloquial speech) or when they cannot be understood by the context, since we are interested in verifying whether intensification features have been maintained in the TT. Formal intensification features are not considered.

Examples:

R.1	VO: ma secondo me, scherzano poi, perche questa costerà un *sacco* di soldi.
	VOSEB: Pero creo que están/bromeando, porque cuestan/*un montón* de dinero.
R.159	VO: E *che* Neruda è catolico. È catolico, lo, lo, *lo so io.*
	VOSEA: Es que Neruda es católico. Es católico, *yo lo sé.*

6.2.4. Morphosyntactic attenuation. These features are informal morphological units and constructions with a minimizing effect. This category includes features of minimization which are typical of oral speech, but also features which can be found in written texts (use of *nosotros* instead of *tú*, diminutive suffixes, indefinite pronouns, adverbs such as *poco*, *nada mal* etc.). These features are typical of colloquial speech, since they minimize the speaker's role in conversation. They are considered in our quantitative study because they cannot be understood from the visual context. Also, it is interesting to observe whether they have been maintained in the TT. Our study does not take into account minimizing features that correspond to courtesy forms, since they are not characteristics of colloquial speech and are much more frequent in formal speech and written texts.

Examples:

R.209	VO: *Uno* si ricorda … "un postino che mi portava la posta quando stavo in Italia"? VD: ¿*Uno* se tiene que acordar del cartero que le llevaba el correo cuando vivía en Italia?
R.4	VO: No. Io so leggere e scrivere, *senza correre*, però … VOSEB: No, sé leer y escribir. *No muy rápido*, pero …

6.2.5. Informal register morphosyntaxis. These structures are typical of colloquial speech, since they either pertain to an informal register or they present an extended meaning and they systematically replace semantically definite expressions. This group also includes expressions which originally pertained to argot but which have lost their socio-cultural connotation over time.

Examples:

R.190	VO: Mo *si mette a parlare* della gente che ha conosciuto. VOSEA: No *va a hablar*/de la gente que conoció.
R.207	VO: Io so' stato a *dare fastidio* a lui. VOSEA: He sido yo quien le ha estado/*dando la lata*.

6.2.6. Tense. This category includes the unconventional use of certain verbal tenses (the use of the present tense to express future or past actions etc.).

Examples:

R.29	VO: Così, quando *prendo* lo stipendio *vado* a Napoli e *faccio vedere* alle ragazze. VOSEB: Así cuando cobre/mi sueldo, *me voy* a Nápoles y se lo *enseño* a las chicas.

6.2.7. Mode. This category includes the unconventional use of verbal modes. This use is quite common in subordinate clauses (the use of the indicative mode instead of the subjunctive or conditional mode etc.) and, if systematic, is an indicator of social dialect.

Examples:

R.170	VO: E pure Voi la *potevate* scrivere allora. VOSEA: Entonces, también Vd./*podía* haberla escrito.

6.3. Lexical features

Lexical features are quite common in colloquial speech and they include three categories:

6.3.1. Informal register lexicon. These lexical units or expressions are more frequent in colloquial speech, since they pertain to informal register. This group includes lexical units with extended meaning which systematically replace semantically definite expressions, as well as lexical units which originally pertained to argot but which have lost their group identity connotation over time.

Examples:

R.148	VO: Lei mi ha messo in questo *guaio*, Lei mi deve tirare fuori. VOSEB: Vd. me metió en este *lío*/y Vd. tiene que sacarme de él.

6.3.2. Vulgar register lexicon. These lexical units and expressions pertain to vulgar register and are more common in colloquial speech. In the following examples only the Italian version presents a swearword (*stronzata*) that could have been translated by an equivalent swearword in Spanish (*gilipollez*). However, all versions translated the swearword by a colloquial expression (*tontería*), which pertains to an informal register and is milder and less offensive that the original term.

Examples:

R.91	VO: Ho detto una *stronzata*, no? VD: Me parece que he dicho una *tontería*. VOSEA: He dicho una *tontería*.

6.3.3. Lexical repetition. This group includes monologic and dialogic repetitions. Monologic repetition is the repetition of (part of) a lexical unit in the same utterance, whilst dialogical repetition is the repetition of a lexical unit which appeared in a previous utterance.

Examples:

R.96	VO: Io so' *innamorato, innamorato proprio, innamorato.* VOSEA: Me he *enamorado, enamorado, /enamorado.*
R.135	*Rosa's bar. Neruda asks Beatrice for a red wine and asks Mario if he also wants red wine:* VO: (*Neruda*) Anche tu un bicchiere di *vino rosso*? (*Mario*) *Vino rosso*, si, anch'io. VOSEC: (*Neruda*) 1– ¿También quieres *vino tinto*? / (*Mario*) – Sí, un *vino tinto.*

6.4. Phonetic features

Within this category, we will confine consideration to pauses, phonetic elongation and phonetic hesitations, since these phenomena, especially the first two, characterize Troisi's idiolect. Tone, frequency, intonation and emphatic pronunciation are not considered, since their analysis would involve the use of instruments such as sonograms and spectrograms.

6.4.1. Phonetic pauses. These are silences in the middle of an utterance and are caused by a lack of planning: speakers doubt how to formulate an utterance since they are unable to choose the correct word or they find it difficult to complete the sentence. Predictable syntactic pauses between utterances and extralinguistic silences caused by external factors are not considered. In the following examples, pauses are represented by a double slash.

Examples:

R.79	VO: No, no, no, no. No la poesia. *Strano // stranoo co' // come* mi sentivo io mentree la dicevate.
	VD: No, no, no. No la poesía. *Extraño // extraño es // cómo* me he sentido yo *mientras // la* recitaba.

6.4.2. Phonetic elongation. It is a relevant elongation of a syllable. Its value is quite similar to that of a pause in the middle of a sentence, since it is related to the speaker's inability to complete the sentence. In the following examples, phonetic elongation is represented by repetition of the vowel, regardless of its duration.

Examples:

R.76	VO: *E chee* che dobbiamo dire noi? Mio padre sì, lui ogni *tantoo* bestemmia *maa* da *soloo*.
	VD: ¿*Queé* qué podemos hacer? Mi padre sí, de vez en *cuandoo* reniega, *peroo paraa* sus adentros.

6.4.3. Loss or addition of sounds. They are generally caused by articulatory relaxation and quick pronunciation (a frequent phenomenon is the loss of –d in the past participle of first conjugation verbs). When this phenomenon is systematic, it is not a colloquial feature but an indicator of social dialect. We do not consider hesitations related to geographic dialect, since they depend on the user and are not colloquial features. In the following examples only the Italian version presents a loss of sounds (*come'l* instead of *come il*).

Examples:

	VO: Co' // *come'l* mare
R.81	VD: Como // *como el* mar
	VOSEB: *Como el* mar.

6.5. Typographic features representing orality

These are orthotypographic elements generally used in subtitling to indicate features such as pauses, omissions, interruptions or to stress the connotation of certain words or expressions, as in the case of argot terms or grammatical mistakes etc. This group includes the use of suspension dots and quotation marks if they imply oral features. A double hyphen (--) is used to indicate oral features in the VOSEC subtitled version distributed in Brazil, but in both versions distributed in Spain this feature is indicated by suspension dots. Interrogative and exclamation marks are excluded, since they are conventional signs used in written texts to represent phonetic elements. Graphic features include two categories:

6.5.1. Suspension dots. These are used to indicate oral features, such as phonetic elongation, anacoluthon, interruptions etc. Suspension dots can be placed at the beginning, at the end or in the middle of a subtitle. It is important to point out that in some subtitled versions (such as VOSEA and, sometimes, VOSEC), suspension dots are systematically used at the end of a subtitle and the beginning of the following subtitle to indicate that the idea was not concluded. In this case, it is not possible to determine whether suspension dots indicate an oral feature and the analysis will only take into consideration suspension dots placed in the middle of a subtitle, at the end of the first line (for two-line subtitles) and at the end of a subtitle if the following subtitle does not include suspension dots at the beginning. Suspension dots can be used in five different cases: to indicate a pause, to underline phonetic elongation, to emphasize interruptions, to emphasize other oral features or to replace colloquial features present in the ST. However, it should be noted that, if the ST is characterized by the simultaneous presence of an interruption, a phonetic elongation and a pause, the suspension points present in the TT will be interpreted as a stressed interruption, since this is their most evident use. For this same reason, if the ST is characterized by the simultaneous presence of a phonetic elongation and a pause, the suspension dots will be interpreted as a stressed pause.

6.5.1.1. Suspension dots indicating pauses which are also present in the ST.

Examples:

R.58	VO: È scritta in aa // straniero.
	VOSEB: Está escrita *en* ... en extranjero.
R.80	VO: *Non soo* // le parole andavano di qua e di là, no?
	VOSEA: *No sé* ... Las palabras iban/de acá para allá.

6.5.1.2. Suspension dots indicating phonetic elongations which are also present in the ST.

Examples:

R.53	VO: *Chee* sta piovendo.
	VOSEB: *Que* ... está lloviendo.
R.141	VO: *Retii*, quali? da ... da pesca?
	VOSEC: *Redes*-- ¿Cuáles redes?/¿Las redes de pesca?

6.5.1.3. Suspension dots emphasizing interruptions which are also present in the ST.

Examples:

R.28	VO: *Io lo dicevo per caso, se* ... // Buon giorno. VOSEA: *No, lo decía por si* ... Buenos días. VOSEC: No, o sea, *si por casualidad*-- Buen día.

6.5.1.4. Suspension dots emphasizing other features: there are no interruptions or phonetic phenomena in the ST. The three dots appear at the end of another colloquial feature in order to reinforce or emphasize it.

Examples:

R.106	VO: Ah, *e lei, e lei* m'ha detto ... VOSEB: *Ella ... Ella* me dijo ... (*Emphasize lexical repetition*)
R.33	VO: *Mario Ruoppolo*, mi chiamo. VOSEB: *Mario Ruoppolo* .../Es mi nombre. (*Emphasize marked order*)

6.5.1.5. Suspension dots replacing other features: they actually replace the colloquial feature present in the ST and are not used to emphasize or reinforce it.

Examples:

R.68	VO: *Pure pure pure* a me mi piacerebbe fare il poeta. VOSEB: *Es que* ... a mí también/me gustaría ser poeta.
R.94	VO: *Vi devo, devo parlare* con Voi, don Pablo. VOSEB: *Debo hablar* ... con Vd./don Pablo.
In both examples, suspension dots replace the lexical repetition present in the ST	

6.5.2. Inverted commas. These are used to emphasize the connotation of certain words or expressions, such as vulgar terms or grammatical errors etc. or to indicate oral features, such as the loss of certain sounds, the use of direct style etc. The conventional use of inverted commas to indicate quotations, bibliographical or literary references, titles of publications etc.

will not be taken into consideration, since this use does not indicate any colloquial features.

Examples:

R.195	VO: Eeh, Don Pablo! ancora // *"Don Pablo ti sentisse".* Don Pablo non mi sente. VOSEA: Otra vez/con *"si te oyera don Pablo".* Don Pablo no me oye.
R.207	VO: Anzi, so' stato io sempre a chiederle: *"Don Pablo, mi correggete sta metafora?" "Don Pablo, mi leggete una poesia?"* VOSEB: Más bien era siempre yo el que le pedía: *"Don Pablo, ¿me corrige esta metáfora? Don Pablo, ¿quiere/leerme esta poesía?"*
R.110	VO: Ee ho detto *"Come ti chiami?"* VOSEC: Le dije, *"¿Cómo te llamas?"*

6.6. Paralinguistic features

These are non-linguistic features. We will confine consideration to symbolic gestures, due to their importance in translation. Our study does not analyse other paralinguistic elements, such as iconic gestures, since their comprehension depends on the context, which is provided by the combination of image, sound and language in a film. Other paralinguistic elements, such as rhythmic gestures or proxemic signs (interpersonal distance, tactile communication) are also discarded because they depend on users and their cultures. Since the purpose of our analysis is to study translation solutions and not cultural differences, these elements will not be considered, given the fact that image cannot be manipulated by translators.

6.6.1. Symbolic gestures. The meaning of these gestures depends on conventions and is unrelated to context. In some cases they are used to emphasize the speaker's words while, in others, they replace speech altogether. This latter case is of special interest for AVT, since these gestures may follow SL conventions and, therefore, are not easily identified or understood by the TL recipient.

Table 2 presents the classification and definition of all the categories proposed in our model of Analysis of Colloquial Informal Speech in AVT.

Table 2: A proposal of categories for the analysis of colloquial informal speech in AVT

Textual organization features
Cohesion with juxtaposition: utterances are linked through juxtaposition, regardless of function (paraphrasing, amplifying, explicating, justifying etc.).
Cohesion with discourse markers: these are markers used in conversation and connectors with an informal or redundant register.
Intensification of discourse markers: these features act as emphasizers in utterances which are linked by discourse markers and stress their meaning.
Cohesion with repetition: utterances are repetitive or redundant and are not linked by connectors: the second utterance has a referential relation to the first one.
Cohesion with pauses: produced when the speaker remains silent for some time before responding to a question, an order, a request etc. or when there is a pause between utterances. Such pauses can be identified as a cohesive feature either because the preceding utterance is incomplete or because the following utterance is redundant (this is not the case of predictable syntactic pauses, which link utterances with a full meaning). Cohesive pauses can be placed before or after a discourse marker or they may even replace it.
Deixis: these features refer to the immediate environment of speech. These features refer to different elements in the immediate or contemporary context or in previous scenes in the film. They can be replaced by the noun they refer to or understood by the context; therefore their use is redundant.
Ellipsis: this textual cohesion procedure is defined by the absence of certain elements in the textual chain. The elided feature can be an utterance, a noun or a verb, although the first case is the most frequent in colloquial speech.
Direct speech: it is a direct discourse in the speech.
Morphosyntactic features
Interruption: anacoluthon, interruption of utterances and involuntary interruptions caused by the speaker.

Marked order: these utterances are characterized by an unconventional word order, with items placed before or after their usual position or with syntactic structures which emphasize certain features by placing them before their usual position.

Morphosyntactic intensification: emphatic or redundant morphological units or informal constructions.

Morphosyntactic attenuation: informal morphological units and constructions with a minimizing effect.

Informal register morphosyntaxis: these structures are typical of colloquial speech, since they either pertain to an informal register or present an extended meaning and systematically replace semantically definite expressions.

Tense: this category includes the unconventional use of verbal tenses

Mode: this category includes the unconventional use of verbal modes.

Lexical features

Informal register lexicon: these lexical units or expressions are more frequent in colloquial speech, since they pertain to informal register. This group includes lexical units which originally pertained to argot and which have lost their group identity connotation over time, as well as lexical units with a broad meaning which systematically replace semantically definite expressions.

Vulgar register lexicon: these lexical units and expressions pertain to the vulgar register and are more common in colloquial speech

Lexical repetition: this group includes monologic and dialogic repetitions. The first one is the repetition of a lexical unit (or a part thereof) in the same utterance; the second one is the repetition of a lexical unit which appeared in a previous utterance.

Phonetic features

Phonetic pauses: a silence in the middle of an utterance. Unlike cohesion pauses, they are due to a lack of planning: the speakers doubt how to formulate an utterance since they are unable to choose the right word or they find it difficult to complete the sentence.

Phonetic elongation: a significant syllabic elongation. Their value is quite similar to that of a phonetic pause.

Loss or addition of sounds: generally caused by articulatory relaxation and quick pronunciation in colloquial speech.

Graphic features
Suspension points: apart from their conventional use, these orthotypographic signs are used to indicate colloquial speech. Suspension points can be used in five different cases: to indicate a pause, to underline phonetic elongation, to emphasize interruptions, to emphasize other oral features or to replace colloquial features present in the source text.
Inverted commas: apart from their conventional use, are used to emphasize the value of certain colloquial words or expressions, such as argot terms or grammatical errors etc. or to indicate oral features, such as the loss of certain sounds, the use of direct style etc.

Paralinguistic features
Symbolic gestures: meaning depends on conventions and is not based on context. In some cases they are used to emphasize the speaker's words while, in others, they replace speech altogether. This latter case is of special interest for AVT since these gestures may follow SL conventions and, therefore, are not easily identified or understood by the TL recipient.

7. Results

Application of this model to our study allowed us to obtain remarkable quantitative and qualitative data. The analysis of such data has led to several conclusions related to the following: (1) the intentionality in the use of colloquial features in the ST; (2) the differences between the ST and its translations in terms of colloquial features; (3) the differences between the use of the different groups of colloquial features depending on the translation mode (dubbing or subtitling); (4) the differences between the use of different categories of colloquial features depending on the translation mode (dubbing or subtitling) (5) the differences between subtitled versions.

(1) Intentionality in the use of colloquial features in the ST.

Table 3: Colloquial features in the ST

Total number of colloquial features: 1361		Total number of exchanges: 218	
What is the distribution of colloquial features in Mario's exchanges?		No.	%
Number of exchanges with colloquial features		197	90.4
Number of exchanges without any colloquial features	Formed by monosyllabs or short syntagms	14	6.4
	Formed by recited poems	7	3.2

Data presented in Table 3 indicates that more than 90% of Mario's exchanges are characterized by informal, colloquial features, regardless of the communicative situation and the protagonist's relation (more or less familiar) to the interlocutor. This percentage is sufficiently relevant to state that the author's purpose was to portray the character from a social point of view.

(2) Differences between the ST and its translations in terms of colloquial features.

Table 4: Presence and absence of equivalent colloquial features in translated versions

VO Features	Features	VD		VOSEA		VOSEB		VOSEC	
1361	Presence	987	72.5%	677	49.7%	708	52%	504	37%
	Absence	374	27.5%	684	50.3%	653	48%	857	63%

All the translated versions are characterized by a relevant reduction of colloquial features compared to the ST (see Table 4). As regards differences between the various translated versions, we can observe that the dubbed version presents a higher percentage of equivalent colloquial features (72.5%), while subtitled version C is the version with the lowest percentage of equivalents (37%). Subtitled versions A and B present around 50%

of informal features (49.7% and 52%, respectively). These data allow us to state that the reduction in the number of colloquial features, both in the dubbed and in the subtitled versions, mirrors the willingness to create more "prepared" oral speech by suppressing oral features and "correcting" non-normative syntactical structures, thus reducing the spontaneity of speech and diminishing Mario's socio-cultural profile. In this sense, none of the translated versions have taken into account the purpose of the colloquial features in the ST, regardless of whether the translation mode was oral (dubbing) or written (subtitling). We can conclude, therefore, that the use of pre-fabricated oral speech does not depend on the translation mode.

(3) Differences in the groups of colloquial features depending on the translation mode (dubbing or subtitling).

The dubbed and subtitled versions make a different use of colloquial features typical of conversation (see Figure 1). Subtitled versions have a more relevant presence of textual organization and morphosyntactic features, whose percentage is higher than in the dubbed version. The latter, on the contrary, presents a high number of phonetic features (greater than 25%).

Figure 1: Groups of colloquial features present in translated versions

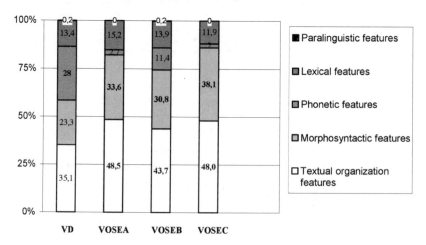

The only category which does not show any meaningful differences is lexical features, whose percentages are quite similar (between 11% and 15%). The presence of phonetic features in the dubbed version and its absence in subtitled versions was predictable. However, while the dubbed version presents a "balanced" distribution of colloquial features in the different categories, for subtitled versions, 70% of these features belong to textual organization and morphosyntactic categories. Therefore, we can conclude that there are substantial differences in the type of colloquial categories used depending on the translation mode.

(4) Differences in the categories of colloquial features depending on the translation mode (dubbing or subtitling).

Translation mode also seems to influence the frequency of colloquial features (see Figure 2). Hence, the most frequent category used in dubbing, in absolute value, is phonetic elongation (17.3%), while the most frequent

Figure 2: Categories of colloquial features present in translated versions

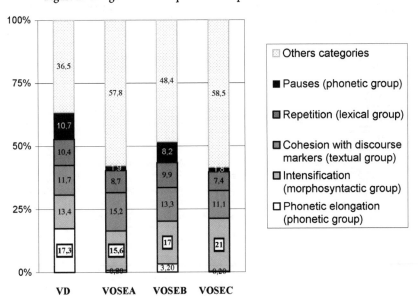

category used in subtitling, in absolute value, is morphosyntactic intensification (15.6%; 17%; and 21%). This data confirms a tendency to use more phonetic features in dubbing and more morphosyntactic features in subtitling and it corroborates the existence of clear differences in the type of colloquial categories used depending on the translation mode.

(5) Differences among subtitled versions.

Table 5: Use of graphic conventions to indicate oral features in subtitled versions

Subtitled versions	Total	Total by uses	Different uses – suspension dots (and double hyphen in VOSEC)
VOSEA	50	13	26% indicate a pause.
		5	10% underline phonetic elongation.
		29	58% stress interruptions.
		3	6% emphasize lexical repetition.
		0	0% replaces colloquial features.
VOSEB	113	58	51.3% indicate a pause.
		23	20.4% underline phonetic elongation.
		22	19.5% stress interruptions.
		5	4.4% emphasize lexical repetition.
		1	0.9% emphasizes marked order.
		3	2.6% replace lexical repetition.
		1	0.9% replaces cohesion with discourse markers.
VOSEC	37	9	24.3% indicate a pause (3/6).
		1	2.7% underline phonetic elongation (0/1).
		27	73% stress interruptions (1/26).
		0	0% replaces colloquial features.

Subtitled versions	Total	Total by uses	Different uses – inverted commas
VOSEA	9	9	100% indicate direct style.
VOSEB	9	9	100% indicate direct style.
VOSEC	8	8	100% indicate direct style.

Data reported in Table 5 reveals that the use of inverted commas is not relevantly different in the three subtitled versions, since frequency is exactly the same and inverted commas are always used to indicate direct style. In this sense, it is interesting to note that inverted commas are not used to indicate oral features, such as argot terms or grammatical errors etc. although orthotypographic conventions would accept this.

The use of suspension dots is relevantly different between subtitled versions. Subtitled version B presents the greatest number of triple dots indicating colloquial features (113), as well as the greatest variety in their use and in the types of colloquial features indicated (they indicate two different types of colloquial features: pauses and phonetic elongation; they reinforce three types of features: interruption, lexical repetition and anticipation; finally, they replace two types of features: lexical repetition and cohesion with discourse markers). Subtitled version C, on the contrary, presents the least number of suspension dots indicating colloquial features (37) and less variety in their use and in the type of feature indicated (pauses and phonetic elongation; they also reinforce interruption and do not replace any types of colloquial feature). Also, version B presents the greatest number of colloquial features in general, while version C presents the least number of such features (Table 4). Therefore, we can conclude that there is a direct relationship between the quantity of orthotypografic signs and the prevalence of colloquial features.

8. Conclusions

From a translational perspective, we believe that our model for the analysis of colloquial informal speech is a valid instrument for the analysis of dubbing and subtitling. Its validation through the pilot study and its application to the analysis of our corpus has allowed us to quantify and describe colloquial features in the source and target texts. The effectiveness of the categories of analysis is revealed by the following aspects:

(1) This model has been designed for translation analysis of dubbing and subtitling. The focus on translation made some of Briz's categories inadequate for our purposes and we, therefore, did not consider them. We have also proposed further categories, which are not considered in Briz's model.

(2) Categories proposed in this model are purely linguistic and concepts such as intention or function have not been considered. This prevents overlapping of different linguistic categories, which were merged in Briz's model. The criteria used in our model makes our categories discrete and mutually exclusive and, therefore, very useful for identifying and describing colloquial informal features.

(3) Categories proposed by this model do not only correspond to linguistic phenomena characteristic of pre-fabricated orality but also to linguistic phenomena derived from colloquial informal speech. This model allows us to examine whether the colloquial features of the source dialogues are deliberately used by the director and whether the translated texts reflect the purpose of the ST by using equivalent colloquial solutions.

(4) This model allows us to undertake comparative analyses between different languages, since it includes linguistic phenomena derived from colloquial informal speech both in Spanish and Italian.

Finally, we believe, that from a methodological point of view, our model for analysing colloquial speech in dubbing and subtitling could be adapted and used to study colloquial speech in different genres or pairs of languages. We also consider that this approach, designed from a translational perspective, could be useful for translators' training. In fact, the variety of categories described allows the development of didactic materials through which the apprentice translator could analyse the different possibilities of representing spontaneous speech in audiovisual translation.

References

Baños, R. (2006), *Estudio descriptivo-contrastivo del español oral en una serie de TV de producción propia y en una serie de TV de producción ajena. El caso de Siete Vidas y Friends.* Master's Thesis, Universidad de Granada.

Bazzanella, C. (1994), *Le facce del parlare. Un approccio pragmatico all'italiano parlato.* Firenze: La Nuova Italia Editrice.

Berretta, M. (1994), Il parlato italiano contemporaneo. In L. Serianni and P. Trifone (eds), *Storia della Lingua Italiana*, vol I, Torino: Einaudi.

Berruto, G. (1985), Per una caratterizzazione del parlato: l'italiano parlato ha un'altra grammatica? In G. Holtus and E. Radtke (eds), *Gesprochenes Italienisch in Geschichte und Gegenwart*, Tübingen: Narr, 120–53.

Briz, A. (1998), *El español coloquial en la conversación. Esbozo de pragmagramática.* Barcelona: Ariel.

Butterworth, B. (1980), Aportaciones del estudio de las pausas en el habla. In Valle et al. (eds), *Lecturas de psicolingüística* 1, Madrid: Alianza, 1990, 289–310.

Chaume, F. (2001), La pretendida oralidad de los textos audiovisuales. In R. Agost and F. Chaume (eds), *La traducción en los medios audiovisuales.* Castelló: Universitat Jaume I.

——(2004), *Cine y traducción.* Madrid: Cátedra.

Coluccia, A. (1996), *Scusate il ritardo. Il cinema di Massimo Troisi*, Torino: Lindau.

Cuenca, M. J. (2008), Pragmatic Markers in Contrast: The Case of Well, *Journal of Pragmatics* 40, 1373–91.

Gregory, M. and S. Carroll (1978), *Language and Situation. Language Varieties and Their Social Contexts.* London: Routledge.

Maclay, H. and C. E. Osgood (1959), Hesitation Phenomena in Spontaneous English Speech, *Word* 15, 19–44.

Mason, I. (1989), Speaker Meaning and Reader Meaning: Preserving Coherence in Screen Translating. In R. Kölmel and J. Payne (eds), *Babel: the Cultural and Linguistic Barriers Between Nations*. Aberdeen: Aberdeen University Press, 13–24.

Matamala, A. (2004), *Les interjeccions en un corpus audiovisual. Descripció i representació lexicogràfica*. PhD Thesis, Universitat Pompeu Fabra.

Poyatos, F. (1980). Interactive Functions and Limitations of Verbal and Non Verbal Behavior in Natural Conversations. *Semiotica* 30, 211–44.

Quilis, A. and C. Hernández Alonso (1990), *Lingüística española aplicada a la terapia del lenguaje*. Madrid: Gredos.

Romero, L. (2010), *Un estudio descriptivo sobre la traducción de la variación lingüística en el doblaje y la subtitulación: las traducciones de Il Postino*. PhD Thesis, Universitat Autònoma de Barcelona.

Romero Fresco, P. (2008), Naturalness in the Spanish Dubbing Language: A Case of not-so-close Friends, *Meta* 59(1), 49–72.

Sabatini, F. (1985), L'italiano dell'uso medio: una realtà tra le varietà linguistiche italiane. In G. Holtus and E. Radtke (eds), *Gesprochenes Italienisch in Geschichte und Gegenwart*. Tübingen: Narr, 154–84.

Sommario, G. (2004), *Massimo Troisi. L'Arte della leggerezza*. Calabria: Rubbettino.

Sacks, H., E. A. Schegloff and G. Jefferson (1974), A Symplest Systematics for the Organization of Turn-taking for Conversation, *Language* 50(4), 696–735.

Televisió de Catalunya (1997), *Criteris lingüístics sobre traducció i doblatge*. Barcelona: Edicions 62.

Valle Arroyo, F. (1991), *Psicolingüística*. Madrid: Eds Morata.

Verardi, C. (1996), *Cinema e palcoscenico: l'universo artistico di Massimo Troisi Tesi di Laurea*. Istituto Universitario Orientale: Napoli. <http://www.netway.it/napoletanità/troisi/tesi/htm/> (accessed 12/2009).

Whitman-Linsen, C. (1992). *Through the Dubbing Glass*. Frankfurt: Peter Lang.

MARIA FREDDI AND SILVIA LURAGHI

Titling for the Opera House:
A Test Case for Universals of Translation?

1. Introduction

Opera titling,[1] that is, the translated lyrics projected above a stage or displayed on a screen, was initially used in opera houses in the 1980s (with the Canadian Opera Company's staging of *Elektra* and the *Meistersinger* at the Maggio Musicale Fiorentino in Florence),[2] gradually becoming more and more common in theatres around the world and partly contributing to the increased popularity of opera (Dewolf, 2001; Mateo, 2007a, 2007b; Orero and Matamala, 2007; Desblache, 2007, 2009).

Within AVT, opera titling is considered a unique type of subtitling as it is used either to transcribe the libretto that may be difficult to understand in the sung form (like intralingual subtitles) or to translate the

---

1   Opera (and more generally theatrical) titles are often referred to as "surtitles" or "supertitles" because of the common practice of projecting them above the stage. However, subtitles shown in individual displays located on the back of seats are becoming increasingly common and are used in leading opera houses, such as the New York Metropolitan Opera, the Royal Opera House at Covent Garden, Milan's Teatro alla Scala, and the Vienna State Opera. For this reason, in this paper we use "titles" and "titling" for all types of operatic sub- and supertitles.

2   The 1986 *Meistersinger* in Florence were titled by Sergio Sablich who organized a Colloquium on translation in music theatre shortly after that ("La traduzione della parola cantata", Florence 12–14 May 1987). The proceedings remain unpublished, but a tape recording is available from the archives of the Teatro del Maggio Fiorentino. See Sablich (2002), Luraghi (2001), and Franchi (2002) for a chronology of opera titling in Italy.

original lyrics into the audience's language (like interlingual subtitles). Unlike cinema subtitles, however, segmentation of titles must consider synchronization with the music as they tend to be launched live, thus retaining an impromptu quality that film subtitles do not have (Mateo, 2002 in Orero and Matamala, 2007: 265; Eugeni, 2006). In addition, titles are more integral to an opera production than film subtitles, as even the single stage interpretation may require changes, adaptations and cuts. They are intrinsic to the staging and dramaturgy and potentially add to the aesthetic and artistic element of opera (Dewolf, 2001; Virkkunen, 2004; Gurewitsch, 2009).

With these assumptions in mind, the present paper sets out to explore translation universals which have been empirically shown to apply to sub-titling for film and television (Gottlieb, 1992 and 1998; Perego, 2005) in order to see whether they also appear as characteristic features of opera titles. The case study chosen for investigation is the English translation of Giuseppe Verdi's operas in the New York Metropolitan Opera ver-sions. In particular, we will analyse Salvatore Cammarano's *Luisa Miller* and Francesco Maria Piave's *La traviata*. The features that emerge from the analysis are further checked against *Aida* titles for opera on film. All three operas considered have been translated by the same translator, Sonya Friedman,[3] so in this regard they are ideal for spotting patterns of linguistic variation in an individual translator's work (Baker, 2004). However, in order to go beyond issues of individual style, examples from titles translat-ing from and into languages other than the Italian-English pair will also be referred to as providing additional evidence for the generalizability of results. The paper aims to research the universals of translation with new evidence, while promoting reflection on a professional practice which is still in its youth.

3   The authors wish to thank Sonya Friedman for allowing them to use her titles.

2. Translation universals in subtitling and surtitling

Translation universals are language features that are found to probabilistically occur in translated texts as a result of the translation/mediation process and are independent of the language pairs involved. It is through large-scale empirical observations of source and target texts (ST and TT) in parallel as well as by comparing translations with non-translated texts that such features have been studied. Because of this, this approach has found in corpora and corpus-based methodology a natural partner, i.e. the Corpus-based Translation Studies which have been welcomed by many as a new paradigm in translatology (Baker, 1993, 1995 and 1996; Laviosa, 2004).

Studies on universals of translation have highlighted simplification and explicitation strategies, normalization and foreignization, then levelling and interference (or transfer), among those most likely to be resorted to by translators. Simplification refers, for example, to the process of reducing lexical repetitions and having recourse to the superordinate term when there are no equivalent hyponyms in the target language (to this extent it overlaps with normalization, see below) and to simplifying complex syntax by replacing it with simpler syntactic structures (e.g. non-finite clauses with finite ones). This two-level process, i.e. lexical and syntactic, will affect the stylistic outcome of the translation, so that it results in stylistic simplification (Laviosa, 1998; Olohan, 2004).

Explicitation on the other hand is the tendency to spell out item relations and parts of the message left implicit in the ST through adding new linguistic material (typically connectives that help to make cohesive relations explicit, interjections and other pragmatic markers that are functional to given characterizations and interpretations, or various kinds of insertions with an explanatory function). Explicitation therefore normally implies an addition, while simplification a subtraction of linguistic items. However, depending on the angle one takes, whether source or target oriented, there may be overlap between the two concepts. Indeed, one can simplify a message without reducing (even extend it) and explicitate without having to add more material, in fact, by reducing some text (Perego 2005: 87–9).

Normalization (also domestication) and the opposite strategy, foreignization, respectively refer to the process of adjusting towards the target
language (TL) and culture or else preserving source language (SL) items
with an estranging effect on the part of the target readership or audience.
Normalization includes replacing old-fashioned expressions with more
modern ones, something which is likely to take place in opera titles, too.
Similarly, levelling indicates the tendency for translated language to con-
verge towards unmarked solutions (as shown, for example, by Kenny's 2001
study of lexical creativity in a corpus of Austrian experimental literature
translated into English). Again, levelling is likely to emerge in librettos
adaptations (Luraghi, 2004; Burton, 2009: 62).

When applied to audiovisual texts and to subtitling procedures, universals have been said to retain specificities linked to the audiovisual mode
of communication and multimodal semiotics (Pérez-González, 2009).
In fact, both simplification and explicitation have been shown to be a
common feature of subtitling (Gottlieb, 1998; Caimi and Perego, 2002;
Perego, 2003; Tomaszkiewicz, 2009) and also present in opera titles with
the aim of facilitating viewers' understanding of the lyrics without preventing them from watching what is happening on stage while listening to the
music (Luraghi, 2004: 16). In this respect, they are often interpretable as
two sides of the same coin aimed at reducing the text processing time on
the part of the viewing audience. Before we consider titles in detail, a brief
overview of Verdi's librettos is in order.

3. Verdi's librettos

Verdi's librettos have been written by different authors; those discussed here,
Luisa Miller, which premiered in 1849, and *La traviata*, premiere 1853, have
been written by Salvatore Cammarano and Francesco Maria Piave respectively, while the libretto for *Aida*, premiere 1871, was written by Antonio
Ghislanzoni. Piave is the most important of Verdi's librettists, because of

the number of librettos he wrote for the composer and his lifelong collaboration with him (Lavagetto, 2003: 65–6). Cammarano is famous for his earlier work with Donizetti; for Verdi he also wrote the libretto for *Il trovatore* which succeeds *Luisa Miller* by a few years (it premiered in the same year as *La traviata*). Antonio Ghislanzoni also collaborated with several composers, including Lauro Rossi, Carlos Gomes and Amilcare Ponchielli; *Aida* is the only libretto he wrote for Verdi. Contrary to *Luisa Miller* and *La traviata*, which were commissioned to Verdi by *impresari* (opera company managers), *Aida* was composed on the occasion of the opening of the Suez Canal, and it was commissioned by the Egyptian khedive Ismail Pasha.

The language of librettos is stylistically marked because of its text-in-music nature; also, it has proven to be highly complex lexically, often convoluted and difficult to disentangle (Baldacci, 1997; Lavagetto, 2003; Bonomi, 2006). Speaking of Verdi's *La traviata*, Baldacci (1997: 93, our translation) remarks that "language, which is always conservative in librettos, here makes one feel that the text has been translated into a dead language".[4] The reason for this is partly to be found in the subject-matter of the drama: "Piave translated concepts which had never before been considered suitable for the heroic world of melodrama" (ibid.; Telve, 1998). The controversial theme of the female protagonist, the prostitute Violetta, had to be concealed by circumlocutions and Latin loans. That similar considerations also hold for *Luisa Miller* is shown by Kallberg's commentary on the 1991 critical edition of the score. Both operas, though differing in many respects, let alone the music, are often compared in the literature. At the time when he was commissioned to write an opera for the Teatro San Carlo in Naples, Verdi had to face censorship problems, something which will also happen with *La traviata* in Venice. The choice of Schiller's drama *Luisa Miller* was dictated by the need to avoid such problems. For this reason, Cammarano eliminated most of the social and political impact of the original text from

---

4   Remarkably, however, colloquial passages can be found in this libretto more than in others, on account of the middle-bourgeois milieu in which the action is set. See Bonomi (2006: 104).

his adaptation; as a result, the intimist drama develops along the more familiar lines and censorship-aware lexical choices of many of Cammarano's earlier librettos.

More importantly, part of the librettos' vocabulary has entered everyday language to become almost idiomatic, which makes it virtually impossible to preserve the lexical creativity and present-day iconicity of the original; see Alfredo's famous aria "De' miei bollenti spiriti / Il giovanile ardore / Ella temprò col placido / Sorriso dell'amore" (*La traviata* act 2 scene 1 "My passionate spirit / and the fire of youth / she tempers with the / gentle smile of love") where the phrase *i miei bollenti spiriti* has crystallized into a fixed expression in Italian (see section 4.1.).

4. Opera titles: A test case for universals of translation?

We can now turn to the analysis of the data chosen for this study. As a general rule, opera titles demand considerable reduction, which is independent of the specific operas (Low, 2002; Luraghi, 2004; Virkkunen, 2004). Nevertheless, space constraints may vary depending on whether one uses surtitles projected over the stage, or subtitles in individual displays. Virkkunen (2004) argues that opera titles either reproduce the verbal-musical complex by expressing in writing the same rhythmic patterns of the original text, or else convey the core contents of the message to facilitate readability and understanding on the part of the audience. This latter strategy can be thought of as a kind of normalization insofar as it is aimed at bringing the libretto closer to the target audience. Virkkunen further stresses how the ST of opera titles is not just the dramatic text, i.e. the score together with the libretto, but also the actual stage interpretation, i.e. each single production of an opera. Such dual nature is likely to affect the type of translation an individual titler might resort to.[5] It must also be noted that opera titles differ from subtitles for opera on film. The latter certainly display similar types of simplification and explicitation; however, their length, segmentation, and omissions crucially depend on the film shooting and individual frames because of the camera close-ups, for example (Burton, 2009: 65).

As already mentioned, according to Baker (1993: 243), universals of translation are "linguistic features which typically occur in translated texts". The combined effects of such universals, which "are thought to be independent of the influence of the specific language pairs involved in the translation process" (ibid.), result in growing standardization, as argued in Toury (1995). Growing standardization is brought about especially by simplification, explicitation, and normalization. In what follows, we will discuss simplification and explicitation in separate sections; normalization will be shown to result from various types of simplification.

4.1. Simplification: Lexical, syntactic and stylistic

4.1.1. Lexical simplification

Lexical simplification is pervasive in opera titles. Indeed, the lexicon of opera librettos is often artificial for reasons partly connected to the specific situational contexts in which librettos have been written, which need not

---

5   Regarding the titles used for this study, the translator has highlighted a difference in the guidelines she received for *Luisa Miller* and *La traviata* remarking that "In *Luisa Miller*, the Met[ropolitan Opera] production was set in an ENGLISH factory-or mill-town, not in a German setting. And the production was quite cool in tone, not reflecting the hot Italian flavour of the libretto. Therefore, the Met requested (strongly!) that I tone down any 'melodrama'. So it was not a question of paraphrasing – it was a question of writing dialogue that those characters singing onstage would have been saying IF they were speaking English, at that (undetermined) time and in a drab, rainy climate. [...] That was not true of *La traviata* – where the Zeffirelli production was traditional" (Sonya Friedman, 2003 p.c.).

concern us here (but see comments in section 3 above). Deviations from
standard lexical choices are usually eliminated from titles. Examples are
numerous, and, in Verdi's librettos (even by different authors), they typically concern a range of words which always occur in place of the standard
equivalent, such as *tempio* [temple] used instead of *chiesa* [church];[6] other
frequent examples are *detto* [said] for *parole* [words], *estinto* [extinguished]
for *morto* [dead], and archaic forms such as *alma* for *anima* [soul] or *egra*
for *malata* [ill]. In some cases, as a result of the simplification process, the
translator even uses words or phrases which are semantically different from
the expression used in the ST:

(1a)   indarno [in vain] / in any case
       (*Luisa Miller* act 2 scene 2)
(1b)   E tutta me pascea [And nourished myself completely] /
       And I would find the answer to life
       (*La traviata* act 1)
(1c)   mistico serto [mystic bough] / source
       (*Aida* act 1 scene 1)

Often, lexical simplification involves lexical periphrases in the ST,
which are removed from the TT. This type of simplification is quite typical of opera titles, as shown in Luraghi (2004: 23–5), and has not been
reported to occur in cinematographic subtitles:

(2a)   il dì che spunta [the day that rises] / today
       (*Luisa Miller* act 1 scene 1)
(2b)   profferse il nome [uttered the name] / named
       (*Aida* act 1 scene 1)
(2c)   Alfredo è in stranio suol [Alfredo is on foreign soil] / Alfredo has
       gone abroad
       (*La traviata* act 3)

---

6   See Baldacci (1997: 96) on the use of this word.

This type of lexical simplification is not restricted to specific pairs of languages, as illustrated in the following examples which involve German as SL and Italian and English as TLs:[7]

(3a) woher *ich kam der Fahrt* / da dove *vengo* / whence *I came*
      (*Lohengrin* act 1 scene 2)
(3b) des Reiches Haupt / sovrano / king
      (*Lohengrin* act 1 scene 2)

Elimination of metonymies and synecdoches can also be considered a type of lexical simplification:

(4a) compra man [a paid hand] / a paid messenger
      (*Luisa Miller* act 2 scene 2)
(4b) queste soglie [this threshold] / this house
      (*Luisa Miller* act 1 scene 3)

Compare, however, the rendering of *soglie* [threshold] in Violetta's aria:

(4c) all'egre soglie ascese [up to the thresholds of sickness he came] / he waited outside my sick *room*
      (*La traviata* act 1)

This process, too, is independent of specific language pairs. In example (5), the metonymy in the Italian text (*i passi miei* [my steps]) is eliminated both from the English and Spanish titles:

---

7   We are of course aware of the enormous difference between Verdi's and Wagner's librettos: for one thing, Wagner wrote the texts for his operas, without resorting to the work of librettists, and the linguistic research behind these texts cannot be compared to the craftsman skills of Verdi's collaborators. However, the degree of lexical complexity in Wagner's texts is comparable if not greater than what we have described for Verdi's librettos, on account, among other things, of the sources used by Wagner, mostly consisting of medieval German poetry (Panagl, 2002).

(5)   seguirai i passi miei / you'll follow me / me seguirás
        (*La traviata* act 2 scene 2)

A shift from the specific to the generic in the TT is sometimes observable, as, for instance, in example (6), where the generic plural noun *possessions* replaces the more specific formulation of the ST (see *cavalli, cocchi* ... [horses, carriages ...]):

(6)   per alienar cavalli, cocchi, / e quanto ancor possiede
        I was selling all my lady's possessions
        (*La traviata* act 2 scene 1)

Lexical simplification can involve compensation. In example (7), the Italian verb *langue* [languish] suggests a state which is not specified by the English verb *be*. However, this lack of expressivity is compensated for by using two adjectives which characterize the referent of the noun phrase *dark, grim prison* as especially bleak and harsh.

(7)   il padre tuo ... langue in dura prigion [your father languishes in a
        hard jail]
        Your father is now in a dark, grim prison
        (*Luisa Miller* act 2 scene 1)

4.1.2. Syntactic simplification

Word order is typically marked in opera librettos and especially so in nineteenth-century melodrama. In titles it usually becomes unmarked for the sake of comprehensibility and clarity rather than fidelity. Note, however, that in the case of translations from Italian into English, the extent to which word order can be freely varied might be thought of as being constrained by systemic differences between the two languages. Nevertheless, the tendency toward normalization of word order goes beyond language-specific constraints, as shown in (8), in which the same order could be preserved in the TT ("Lovely is the April dawn, but ..."):

(8) leggiadra è quest'alba sorgente in aprile,
     ma come il tuo viso, leggiadra no, non è [graceful is this rising dawn
     in April,/but like your face, graceful no, it is not]
     The April dawn is lovely,
     but no lovelier than your face.
     (*Luisa Miller* act 1 scene 1)

In (9), the recovery of the unmarked word order has an effect of thematizing Luisa's self-denial with the consequent shift in focus on *for me*, i.e. the higher moral value for which she has renounced Rodolfo:

(9) All'amor tuo per me rinunziasti. [Your love for me you gave up]
     You sacrificed your true love for me
     (*Luisa Miller* act 3 scene 1)

In addition, as shown in (10), even a much closer TL as Spanish to Italian most often presents normalized orders (note also lexical simplification, consisting in the omission of the adjectives *segrete* [secret] and *amico* [friendly]):

(10) le cure segrete / fuga sempre l'amico licor
      ¡El licor ahuyenta las penas!
      (*La traviata* act 1)

That normalization of word order is not language specific is also shown by the following examples, where the SL is German and the TL Italian:

(11a) verloren ist dein Leben [lost is your life] / la tua vita è perduta!
       (*Die Zauberflöte* act 1)
(11b) und ewig wäre sie dann mein [and forever would she then be mine]
       / sarebbe mia, per sempre
       (*Die Zauberflöte* act 1)[8]

---

8 These examples are discussed by Grizzo (2005) who also shows cases in which the translated text maintains the German marked word order.

Syntactic simplification operates on more than just one level, e.g. word order, and often involves full restructuring of the ST syntax, as, for instance, in (12) below:

(12)   Un angiol che in esilio quaggiù mandava il ciel. [an angel whom in exile down here the heavens sent]
An angel in exile, sent here by Heaven ...
(*Luisa Miller* act 3 scene 1)

Among other types of syntactic simplification, we must mention frequent changes in the diathesis, whereby the passive and middle voice is changed into active:

(13a)   l'opra mia si compia [my work be completed]/ I must fulfill my task
(*Luisa Miller* act 2 scene 2)
(13b)   Poiché dal ciel non furono tai nodi benedetti ... [Because from the heavens were not such ties blessed]
For Heaven cannot bless a union such as this
ya que el cielo no bendijo vuestra unión
(*La traviata* act 2 scene 2)
(13c)   er ist befreit durch unseres Armes Tapferkeit [he is freed thanks to our arm's bravery]
il nostro coraggio lo ha liberato
(*Die Zauberflöte* act 1)
(13d)   Verwirrung, wilde Fehde wird mir kund [Confusion, wild revenge became known to me]
I hear confusion and strife
vedo disordine ovunque, ostilità
(*Lohengrin* act 1 scene 1)

However, the change also happens in the opposite direction, from active into passive, especially when involving a switch from marked to unmarked word order, as in (14):

(14) De' miei bollenti spiriti / Il giovanile ardore
Ella temprò col placido / Sorriso dell'amore! [of my boiling spirits,
the youthful ardour/She calmed with the serene smile of love]
The tempestuous urgency / Of my youthful passion ...
... has been calmed / by her gentle smile ...
(*La traviata* act 2 scene 1)

It is clear from the last example how several changes and adaptations occur simultaneously (not just the passive, but also recovery of the unmarked constituent order, not to mention lexical variation), each contributing to the overall normalizing and simplification tendency. This leads us onto the next issue of stylistic simplification.

4.1.3. Stylistic simplification

The cases discussed so far, exemplifying lexical and syntactic simplification, also result in stylistic simplification. In the next example, lexical simplifications are accompanied by elimination of rhyme:

(15) Fra' mortali ancora oppressa / non è tanto l'innocenza, che si vegga genuflessa / d'un superbo alla presenza [Among mortals not yet so oppressed/is innocence/that it is seen kneeling in the presence of arrogance]
Innocence is not yet so oppressed that it must kneel before arrogance
(*Luisa Miller* act 1 scene 2)

As far as stylistic simplification is concerned, sometimes full lines are omitted or condensed. This procedure has been found to occur systematically in concertato numbers, i.e. when three or more characters sing together, each overlapping with their lines. Concertatos involve repetition of the same verses, which is avoided in opera titles; therefore omission and condensation are recurrent. An example is provided by the finale of the first act of *Luisa Miller*:

(16a) WALTER: Il mio cenno, il voler mio / è immutabil come il fato!
LUISA: Ad immagin tua creata, / o Signore, anch'io non fui? / E
perché son calpestata / or qual fango da costui? / Perché? perché? /
Deh, mi salva... deh, m'aita... / deh! non m'abbia l'oppressor! / Il
tuo dono, la mia vita / pria riprenditi, Signor!
MILLER: A quel Dio ti prostra innante, / de' malvagi punitor, / non
a tal che ha d'uom sembiante, / e di belva in petto il cor.
RODOLFO: Cedi all'amor mio, / ah padre, cedi! / Negro vel mi sta
sul ciglio! / Ho l'inferno in mezzo al cor! / Un istante ancor son
figlio! / Un instante ho padre ancor!
WALTER: Piegarti devi, non io, / o figlio ingrato. / Fra il suo core e
il cor paterno / frapponeste un turpe amor. / Non può il ciel, non
può l'inferno / involarvi al mio furor!
LAURA, SOME PEASANTS: Il suo pianto al pianto sforza! / Il suo
duolo spezza il cor!
ALCIERI: Obbedirlo a tutti è forza! / Egli è padre, egli è signor!
WALTER: I cenni miei si compiano.

which is condensed as follows:

WALTER: My will is as unchangeable as fate!
LUISA: Oh Lord, was I not also created in Your image? Then why
am I trampled into the mud by this man? Help me, save me from
this oppressor or else take back the gift of my life, Lord.
WALTER: See that my orders are carried out.
(*Luisa Miller* act 1 scene 2)

See also the end of scene 2 in the second act; it is again the concertato
that entails stylistic simplification and omission in the TT:

(16b) (Pinto ha di vivo giubilo / il sorridente viso!
Fortuna in quel sorriso / propizia balenò!
Ben io fermarla, e stringerne / l'infido crin saprò.)
Our fortune is secure
now that the noble lady smiles!
(*Luisa Miller* act 2 scene 2)

Duets, on the other hand, because of the tight rhythm, may be condensed in a smaller number of turns, as in (17):

(17) VIOLETTA: Questi luoghi abbandonate, / un periglio vi sovrasta ...
ALFREDO: Ah comprendo! / Basta ... basta ... / E sì vile mi credete? ...
VIOLETTA: Ah, no, mai ...
ALFREDO: Ma che temete?
VIOLETTA: Leave this place, you're in danger.
ALFREDO: I understand you think I'm a coward.
(*La traviata* act 2 scene 2)

Ultimately, the extent to which entire verses or parts thereof are omitted in opera titles seems to depend on individual translators (Virkkunen, 2004). Compare the following examples, in which the SLs are Italian and German, and the TLs are English, Finnish, Spanish, French, Dutch and Italian:

(18a) Amami, Alfredo. Amami quant'io t'amo.
Love me, Alfredo. Love me as much as I love you.[9]
Love me, Alfredo. Love me as I love you.[10]
Rakasta minua niin kuin minä rakastan sinua [Love me as much as I do][11]
(*La traviata* act 1)
(18b) D'Alfredo il padre, la sorte, l'avvenir
domanda or qui De' suoi due figli ...
I ask you to decide the fate of both my children
El padre de Alfredo ha venido a pediros por la suerte de sus dos hijos
[Alfred's father has come beg you for the fate of his two sons]
(*La traviata* act 2 scene 1)

---

9 Cited in Virkkunen (2004: 11).
10 Sonya Friedman's titling.
11 Cited in Virkkunen (2004: 90).

(18c) Hi! Ho! Waldhüter ihr, Schlafhüter mitsammen, so wacht doch
       mindestens am Morgen!
       Hé! Gardes du bois! Veillez au moins ò l'aurore!
       Bewakers van het woud, hoeders van de slaap word toch wakker[12]
       [Guards of the forest, guardians of sleep do wake up]
       (*Parsifal* act 1)

(18d) Hört! Grafen, Edle, Freie von Brabant! Heinrich, der Deutschen
       König, kam zur Statt, mit euch zu dingen nach des Reiches Recht.
       Hear ye, nobles and freemen of Brabant / Heinrich, King of Germany,
       comes here to confer with you as the law request
       Nobili di Brabante! Il re dei tedeschi, Heinrich, è venuto a conferire
       con voi.
       (*Lohengrin* act 1 scene 1)

Peripheral linguistic items such as interjections, exclamations, expletives (*ah!*, *oimè*, *oh Dio*, *oh ciel* etc.) and other pragmatic markers, such as
vocatives, are often eliminated in titles, something which has been shown to
hold true of subtitling in general (Tomaszkiewicz, 2009). In (19) the inter-
jection *deh* is eliminated both from the English and Spanish titles; the latter
then goes one step further by also eliminating the vocative *Violetta*:

(19) Violetta, deh, pensateci, Ne siete in tempo ancor!...
      Violetta, think about it. There's still time
      Pensad en ello, todavía estáis a tiempo
      (*La traviata* act 2 scene 1)

In the following excerpt from *Luisa Miller*, the translator omits Miller's
last line completely, which leaves the singing isochronous with his gesture
unfilled by the translation.[13] The line "Che foglio è questo" is completely
omitted after the shortened aside:

---

12   Cited in Dewolf (2001: 183).
13   In discussing film subtitling, Tomaszkiewicz (2009: 25) argues that redundancy
     between the visual and the verbal codes is one of the prerequisites for any manipula-
     tion of the original text and specifically for omissions and condensations.

(20) (Quella calma è funesta!
Il cor mi serra non so qual rio presagio!)
[takes the letter]
Che foglio è questo?
(This calm of hers is dangerous. I feel it in my heart.)
(*Luisa Miller* act 3 scene 1)

In the same scene between Luisa and her father, the following lines are completely eliminated from the English version by Sonya Friedman, probably because the reconciliation is conveyed by the kinesics together with the next turn, which conversely gets translated in the title (cf. Ah! in quest'amplesso l'anima oblia quanti martiri provò finor / with this embrace, let our souls forget all past suffering):

(21) MILLER: Figlia?
LUISA: La figlia, vedi, pentita / al piè ti cade.
MILLER: No, figlia mia, / sorgi, qui sul mio cor.
LUISA: Padre, ah, mio padre!
(*Luisa Miller* act 3 scene 1)

A form of stylistic simplification that we found in the titles of the TV version of *Aida* concerns the condensation of two turns belonging to different characters into one, as observable in (22). This is possibly due to the fact that the camera has a close-up on *Aida*:

(22) MESSAGGERO: Un guerriero / indomabile, feroce / li conduce
– Amonasro
TUTTI: *Il re!*
AIDA: (Mio padre!)
MESSENGER: An indomitable warrior leads them – *King* Amonasro
AIDA: (My father)
(*Aida* act 1 scene 1)

Stylistic simplification can also consist of the elimination of metaphors.[14] In the following example, the ST contains a metaphor by which the illness (*la tisi* [tubercolosis]) is conceived as an agent. In the titles, the metaphorical phrasing is removed, to the effect that the only mention of Violetta's illness is suppressed, with a consequent loss of information:

(23) la tisi non le accorda che poche ore [consumption only gives her a
      few hours]
      she has only a few more hours to live
      (*La traviata* act 3)

In conclusion, an overall tendency towards normalization and register levelling is observable in the data under study, as a consequence of the simplification processes at work in translation. As becomes clear from the examples discussed, figures of speech are usually levelled out and so are syntactic ornaments. As mentioned in section 3, the lowering of the register is inevitable, due to the poetic nature and farfetched quality of much of the language of the librettos examined (Low, 2008; Burton, 2009). Compare the following two examples:

(24a) Ad ottenerlo, contaminato / mi son purtroppo di *nero eccesso*! [To
      obtain it, I unfortunately covered myself of a black excess]
      But to obtain it, I committed *a terrible crime*
      (*Luisa Miller* act 2 scene 2)
(24b) *Tutto è follia* nel mondo / Ciò che non è piacer. [all is madness in
      the world,/Which is not pleasure]
      Nothing in the world *matters* / Except pleasure
      (*La traviata* act 1)

Notice the lowering effect of the shift in the negation and the suppression of the word *follia* [folly].

---

14   Indeed, removal of metaphors is more than simply stylistic simplification, involving
     the elimination of the conceptual shift necessary for the listener/reader to process
     the metaphor.

4.2. Explicitation: Linguistic and cultural

Translated texts ostensibly display a higher level of explicitness with respect to their STs, as argued by various authors (Baker, 1995; Laviosa, 1998: 289; Olohan, 2004: 92–6). Explicitation can operate on the linguistic level, for example by replacing ellipses with full forms or indirect with direct references, as well as on the cultural level, the latter often occurring in the form of domestication.

4.2.1. Linguistic explicitation

In the following example, while the original line relies on extra-linguistic reference, i.e. on information that can be retrieved from the situational context, because of the props on stage, the title opts for linguistic redundancy:

(25) RODOLFO [showing him two guns]
Scegliere tu dèi. [Choose you must]
Choose *your weapon*
(*Luisa Miller* act 2 scene 3)

In example (26), the generic demonstrative *quel* is amplified as "that chosen" to help identify the referent:

(26) Se *quel* guerrier io fossi!
If only I were *that chosen* warrior!
(*Aida* act 1 scene 1)

whereas in (27) the same demonstrative is replaced by a possessive noun phrase, again explicitating the identity of the referent:

(27) non era muto ancor *quel* labbro! [It was not mute yet that lip]
The *old man's* lips were not yet silent
(*Luisa Miller* act 2 scene 2)

Notice the expansion in (28), in which Alfredo's allusion to Violetta's conditions in the ST is made explicit (cf. *in cotal guisa* [in that guise]:

(28) Ah, *in cotal guisa* / V'ucciderete ...
      This life you lead will kill yourself
      (*La traviata* act 1)

In general, compact noun phrases are unpacked into more explicit verbal phrasings: see, for example, *Oh mio rimorso! Oh infamia!* rendered as "I've disgraced my self!" and *la vita è nel tripudio* turned into "we live only for pleasure", both from *La traviata*, the latter with the explicitating addition of "only", and *lo sguardo innamorato* rendered as "gaze lovingly" in (29):

(29) ... meco figgea nell'etere / lo sguardo innamorato,
      ... she and I would gaze lovingly / at the heavens
      (*Luisa Miller* act 2 scene 3)

Explicitation can take the form of a real dénouement, as in the next example, where the title anticipates the target of Radames's love by spelling out the obscure *arcano amore* [arcane love] with "I love her slave":

(30) (Forse ... l'arcano amore / Scoprì che m'arde in core ...)
      (can she suspect that I love her slave?)
      (*Aida* act 1 scene 1)

In (31) from *La traviata*, the explicitation process has a complex shape because of the multiple syntactic changes, that is, the embedded structure with the relative clause is unpacked into two juxtaposed independent clauses (Stampacchia, 2004: 88), the first person singular subject pronoun replaces *l'amor* [love] and is repeated twice as a result of the juxtaposition, and the deictic "(for) you" is added:

(31) *L'amor* che m'ha guidato, / Sa tutto perdonar. [The love which guided me/Can everything forgive]
      I came here out of love *for you* / *I* forgive *you* for everything
      (*La traviata* act 2 scene 1)

This happens also in Violetta's aria at the end of the first act when she sings:

(32) E tutta me pascea / *Di quel divino error.*
      [And nourished myself completely / On that divine error]
      And I would find the answer to life / in *my passion for him.*
      (*La traviata* act 1)

where the indirect reference of the distal demonstrative becomes the first person possessive adjective "my" and the "divine error" is again spelled out as "passion for him".

Words might also be added to better qualify the topic, as in *l'amor tuo* [your love] / "your true love" (*Luisa Miller* act 3 scene 1), or in example (33) from Rodolfo's aria:

(33) Se cielo e terra, se mortali ed angeli attestarmi volesser ch'ella non è rea, mentite! [If heavens and earth, if mortals and angels wanted to assure me that she is not guilty, you lie!]
      [showing the letter]
      If Heaven, earth, mortals and angels *all* assured me she was not guilty
      (*Luisa Miller* act 2 scene 3)

In the party scene from *La traviata*, example (34), the insertion of the adjective "exotic" contributes to the characterization of the atmosphere created by the ballet number of the gypsies and matadors:

(34) Noi siamo zingarelle / Venute da lontano [We are gipsy women / Come from afar]
      We're gypsies from / a far-off, *exotic* land
      (*La traviata* act 2 scene 2)

In example (35) the noun phrase *dovizie, amori e le pompose feste* is explicitated by being first referred to by a collective expression "everything and everyone" then unpacked in "a life of wealth, fame and lavish parties":

(35)   Dacché la mia Violetta / Agi per me lasciò, dovizie, amori
       E le pompose feste / Ove, agli omaggi avvezza,
       Vedea schiavo ciascun di sua bellezza [Since my Violetta/Wealth for
       me left, abundance, love/And the lavish parties/Where to compi-
       ments accustomed,/She saw everyone as slave to her beauty]
       Violetta left everything and everyone for me
       A life of wealth, fame and lavish parties ...
       ... where every man was a slave to her beauty
       (*La traviata* act 2 scene 1)

Even famous arias, where the text has become as iconic as the music itself,
present instances of explicitation in the titles. This is well exemplified by
the last part of Alfredo's aria "Un dì felice ..." culminating with the expression *croce e delizia al core*, which in the English text shows various kinds of
shifts, amplifications and even repetition:

(36)   E da quel dì tremante vissi / D'ignoto amor
       Di quell'amor ch'e' palpito / Dell'universo intero,
       Misterioso, altero, / Croce e delizia al cor. [Since that day trembling
       I lived/Of unknown love/Of love that is the pulse/Of the entire
       universe,
       Mysterious, proud,/Cross and delight of the heart]]
       Since then I've adored you in secret
       My whole being throbs with love
       A love that fills the entire universe
       Never have I known such a mysterious force
       Such pain! Such delight! Such heartfelt delight.
       (*La traviata* act 1)

Sometimes, explicitation works through a hendiadys, whereby a subordinat-
ing pair comprised of an adjective modifying a noun is transformed into
two coordinating nouns, *il mio rigor crudele* [my cruel rigour] / "my cruelty
and severity", or, as in (37), when the adjective *dura* [tough] is unpacked
into two coordinating elements:

(37)   in dura prigion / in a dark, grim prison
       (*Luisa Miller* act 2 scene 1)

Contrary to lexical simplification as discussed in relation to shifts from specific to generic (section 4.1.1.), an explicitating tendency is to be found in the use of concrete nouns in preference to abstract ones, as is observable in the pairs *amistà* [friendhip] / "your friends" (also, "good friends" as found in *La traviata*) and the specific in lieu of the generic, as in *il foglio* [the sheet] / "the letter", and *per goder* [to have fun] becoming "for the next party".

A special type of translation strategy which, as far as we can tell, seems typical of opera titles concerns personal deixis. Often, in Verdi's librettos, a character refers to him-/herself in the third person, through noun phrases like *tua figlia* [your daughter], *il padre* [the father], *l'amica* [the friend], *un genitor* [a parent] etc. In the English titles, first and second person personal pronouns are often introduced in such cases to replace the indirect reference:

(38a)   Taci! Uccider vuoi *tua figlia*? [Quiet! Do you want to kill your daughter?]
        Quiet, do you want to kill *me*?
        (*Luisa Miller* act 1 scene 3)
(38b)   *D'Alfredo il padre*, la sorte, / l'avvenir domanda or qui de' suoi due figli [Alfred's father, the fate,/the future demands now here/of his two children]
        I ask you to decide / the fate of both my children
        (*La traviata* act 2 scene 2)

Or, in the same scene between Violetta and Germont:

(38c)   E' Dio che ispira, o giovane, / tai detti *a un genitor* [It is God who suggests, oh young one,/such sayings to a parent]
        God himself inspires this plea *of mine*
        (*La traviata* act 2 scene 2)

The indirect reference in the original librettos stereotypically pointing to the roles and relationships between characters is replaced with a personal pronoun in the translation. This way, from the point of view of the text processing time and effort, personal deixis is most clearly expressed with no mismatch between speaker and interlocutors' roles and the first and second person pronouns used to lexicalize them (*I/me, you*). Note, however, that there are also cases in which the third person reference is preserved in the title, so it is difficult to identify any regularity there. Again in *La traviata*, Germont says to Alfredo:

(39a) Ritorna *di tuo padre* orgoglio e vanto [Be again your father's pride and yoy]
Be *your father's* pride and joy again
(*La traviata* act 2 scene 2)

And from *Luisa Miller*:

(39b) T'arrendi a me, / tradirti *il padre tuo*, no, non può [Surrender to me,/betray you your father cannot]
Put your trust in me
Your father could never betray you
(*Luisa Miller* act 2 scene 3)

In the last example, taken from an exchange between Walter, Rodolfo's father, and his son, the literal translation in the title preserves the dramatic effect of the original (how could a father betray his son?). Similar examples of preservation are also numerous in act 2 from *La traviata* between Alfredo and Germont as well as in *Aida*.

Analogously, possessives are added to avoid referential confusion:

(40a) Ben la conobbe il padre [Well knew her the father]
My father was right about her
(*Luisa Miller* act 2 scene 3)

(40b) *Del genitore*, oh quanto caro / lo scampo a te costava! [from the
  father, oh how dear/the release cost you]
  How dearly you've paid for *your father's* release
  (*Luisa Miller* act 3 scene 1)
(40c) Ah! nella tomba che schiuder vuoi
  fia primo a scendere *il genitor*!
  Then let *your father* descend
  into the tomb you would open!
  (*Luisa Miller* act 3 scene 1)

Convergence on the personal pronoun most directly lexicalizing the referent can be seen also in example (40d):

(40d) Se mia foste, custode io veglierei / pe' *vostri soavi dì* [if you were
  mine, like a guardian I would watch/over your pleasant days]
  If you were mine I'd watch over *you*
  (*La traviata* act 1 scene 1)

Along the same lines, indirect references are repeatedly explicitated through
the TT recovery of the nominal head for the referent of the adjectival
construction, see *l'infelice* [the unhappy] / "the poor girl", and *l'infame* [the
wicked] / "the vile woman", and also *empio* [evil] / "evil man" (all from
Luisa Miller). In (41) the understated form *la traviata* [the debauched]
with which the protagonist refers to herself is replaced with the more direct
expression "this lost woman". While this change certainly results in explicitation (note also the addition of the proximal demonstrative "this"), it also
has the effect of losing the iconicity of Violetta's self-reference through the
designation that serves as title for the opera:

(41) Ah, *della traviata* sorridi al desio [Ah, smile at the depraved woman's
  desire]
  Grant *this lost woman* one final wish
  (*La traviata* act 3)

Explicitation through addition of linguistic material to obtain further specification can also be seen in:

(42) E sdegnar*la* poss'io ...? [And can I ignore it ...?]
      Can I ignore *such a chance* ...?
      (*La traviata* act 1).

(43) O dolce amica, e ristorar non vuoi di qualche cibo le affralite membra?
      [Oh sweet friend, don't you want to refresh/With some food the
      ailing limbs?]
      Sweet friend, won't you take some food to refresh yourself?
      (*Luisa Miller* act 3 scene 1)

In example 43 above, lexical simplification combines with explicitation, the former concerning substitution of the metonymy *affralite membra* [weakened limbs] with "yourself", while the latter involves the unpacking of *ristorar di qualche cibo* [refresh with some food] into the explicit subordination between the two clauses "take some food to refresh".

4.2.2. Cultural explicitation

Cultural explicitation occurs when homophoric references, unless explicitated, may be vague or jeopardize understanding on the part of the viewer, as for instance in 44–6 (cf. the explicitating shift from *Re* [King] to "Pharao", or *un Giusto, un Possente* [a Righteous, a Mighty] becoming "Righteous God":

(44) *La sacra Iside* consultasti? [Did you consult the sacred Isis?]
      Have you consulted *our sacred goddess Isis*?
      (*Aida* act 1 scene 1)

(45) Ora del Nume / reco i decreti *al Re* [Now the Goddess' decrees/I
      bring to the king]
      I shall inform *the Pharao* of the goddess decree
      (*Aida* act 1 scene 1)

(46) Havvi un Giusto, un Possente / che il guardo tien rivolto sui miseri ognor! [Is there a Just, a Powerful/who keeps an eye on the wretched all the time?]
Righteous God always watches over the wretched
(*Luisa Miller* act 2 scene 2)

Culture-specific terms, including idiomatic expressions, present changes from specific to more easily recognisable references for the target audience, as in (47), in which the name of a single classical deity, though appropriate for a toast (according to Greek mythology Ebe was the goddess who poured wine during the gods' banquets on Olympus and not one of the Muses), is replaced with the more easily identifiable "muse", which refers to a group of deities known for inspiring artists, thus equally appropriate for a toast:

(47) Sarò l'Ebe che versa [I will be the Hebe who pours]
Am I *his muse*?
(*La traviata* act 1)

This kind of shift, which clearly is a form of domestication, also affects idiomatic expressions, as observed in (48), where the aphoristic formulation of the original is maintained through an equivalent saying in the TL:

(48) La volpe lascia il pelo. Non abbandona il vizio [A fox sheds its fur. It does not foresake vice]
A leopard can't change its spots
(*La traviata* act 2 scene 2)

5. Conclusions

In this paper we have examined some translational strategies in titling for opera and have questioned whether opera titles could be a test case for universals of translation as described to pertain to other translation modes and genres both within AVT and beyond. In order to respond, we considered three operas by Giuseppe Verdi, titled in English, by the same translator and compared the results with translations involving different language pairs and librettos from different periods and stylistic preferences (e.g. Mozart's and Wagner's). Analysis has shown the pervasiveness of some features, e.g. lexical, syntactic and stylistic simplification as well as linguistic and cultural explicitation (see, for instance, the recovery of syntactic linearity in examples 8–12).

Genre-specificities have emerged within the universal tendencies described in the literature concerning the extent of lexical and stylistic simplification as well as linguistic explicitation, which seem to be higher than in other genres. In particular, tendency to replace lexical periphrases with simpler lexical items (section 4.1.1.) and substitution of direct for indirect deixis (section 4.2.1.), which are highly recurrent in our corpus, seem to be specific to opera titles. However, individual translator's choices may affect the frequency of resorting to these strategies, as well as opera companies imposing their own house style (Burton 2009: 64). The degree to which variation and regularity across translations of titles can be observed thus covers the whole gamut, from virtually no paraphrasing, as in the Teatro alla Scala's literary translations given in the subtitles, tellingly called "electronic librettos",[15] to high stylistic simplification and rephrasing in the titles analysed.

---

15   Indeed the use of full translations, which are adapted only for musical purposes (i.e. title cuts are decided depending on the music and timing of what is going on on stage) rather than comprehension is a common practice in several Italian opera houses, not just La Scala, as confirmed by Mauro Conti of Prescott Studio, one of the few independent producers of titles for the stage in Italy (see <http://www. prescott.it>; accessed 01/10/2010).

References

Baker, M. (1993), Corpus Linguistics and Translation Studies: Implications and Applications. In M. Baker, G. Francis and E. Tognini Bonelli (eds), *Text and Technology. Studies in Honour of John Sinclair*. Amsterdam: John Benjamins, 233–50.

—— (1995), Corpora in Translation Studies: an Overview and some Suggestions for Future Research. *Target* 7(2), 223–43.

—— (1996), Corpus-based Translation Studies: The Challenges that Lie Ahead. In H. Somers (ed.), *Terminology, LSP and Translation. Studies in Language Engineering in Honour of Juan C. Sager*. Amsterdam: John Benjamins, 175–86.

—— (2004), A Corpus-based View of Similarity and Difference in Translation. *International Journal of Corpus Linguistics* 9(2), 167–93.

Baldacci, L. (1997), *La musica in italiano*. Milano: Rizzoli.

Bonomi, I. (2006), La lingua dell'opera lirica. In P. Trifone (ed.), *Lingua e identità. Una storia sociale dell'italiano*. Roma: Carocci, 87–112.

Burton, J. (2009), The Art and Craft of Opera Surtitling. In J. Díaz-Cintas and G. Anderman (eds), *Audiovisual Translation: Language Transfer on Screen*. London: Palgrave Macmillan, 58–70.

Caimi, A. and E. Perego (2002), Sottotitolazione: lo stato dell'arte. *RILA– Rassegna Italiana di Linguistica Applicata* 34 (1–2), 19–51.

Desblache, L. (2007), Music to my Ears, but Words to my Eyes? Text, Opera and their Audiences. *Linguistica Antverpiensia. New Series –Themes in Translation Studies* 6, 155–70.

—— (2009), Challenges and Rewards of Libretto Adaptation. In J. Díaz-Cintas and G. Anderman (eds), *Audiovisual Translation: Language Transfer on Screen*. Basingstoke: Palgrave Macmillan, 71–82.

Dewolf, L. (2001), Surtitling Operas with Examples from Translations from German into French and Dutch. In Y. Gambier and H. Gottlieb (eds), *(Multi)Media Translation: Concepts, Practices, Research*. Amsterdam: John Benjamins, 179–88.

Eugeni, C. (2006), Il sopratitolaggio: definizione e differenze con il sottotitolaggio. *IntraLinea* 8. <http://www.intralinea.it/volumes/ita_more.php?id=259_0_2_0_C> (accessed 05/07/2010).

Franchi, S. (2002), Leggere l'aria. *Il Giornale della Musica*, 181.

Gottlieb, H. (1992), Subtitling: A New University Discipline. In C. Dollerup and
    A. Loddegaard (eds), *Teaching Translation and Interpreting*, vol 1. Amsterdam:
    John Benjamins, 161–70.
——(1998), Subtitling. In M. Baker (ed.), *Routledge Encyclopedia of Translation Studies*.
    London: Routledge, 244–8.
Grizzo, S. (2005), *Il traduttore all'opera: Analisi dei sopratitoli de* Die Zauberflöte *di
    W. A. Mozart*. Unpublished MA Thesis, University of Trieste.
Gurewitsch, M. (2009), Entitlement Issues. *Opera News* 74, 38–9.
Kallberg J. (1991), *Introduction to* Luisa Miller *by Giuseppe Verdi. Critical Edition*.
    Chicago: Chicago University Press and Milan: Ricordi, vii–xiv.
Kenny, D. (2001), *Lexis and Creativity in Translation: A Corpus-based Study*.
    Manchester: St. Jerome.
Lavagetto, M. (2003), *Quei più modesti romanzi. Il libretto nel melodramma di Verdi*.
    Torino: EDT.
Laviosa, S. (1998), Universals of Translations. In M. Baker (ed.), *Routledge Encyclopedia
    of Translation Studies*. London: Routledge, 288–91.
——(2004), Corpus-based Translation Studies: Where Does it Come From? Where
    Is it Going? *Language Matters* 35(1), 6–23.
Low, P. (2002), Surtitles for Opera: A Specialised Translating Task. *Babel* 48(2),
    97–110.
——(2008), Translating Songs that Rhyme. *Perspectives: Studies in Translatology*
    16(1–2), 1–20.
Luraghi, S. (2001), Canta che ti passa: il sopratitolo. *Classic Voice* 27, 52–5.
——(2004), Sottotitoli per l'opera: strategie di semplificazione in un tipo speciale
    di traduzione. *SILTA – Studi Italiani di Linguistica Teorica e Applicata* 33(1),
    27–48.
Mateo, M. (2007a), Reception, Text and Context in the Study of Opera Surtitles.
    In Y. Gambier, M. Schlesinger and R. Stolze (eds), *Doubts and Directions in
    Translation Studies*. Amsterdam: John Benjamins, 169–82.
——(2007b), Surtitling Today: New Uses, Attitudes and Developments. *Linguistica
    Antverpiensia. New Series* 6, 135–54.
Olohan, M. (2004), *Introducing Corpora in Translation Studies*. London:
    Routledge.
Orero, P., and A. Matamala (2007), Accessible Opera: Overcoming Linguistic and
    Sensorial Barriers. *Perspectives: Studies in Translatology* 15(4), 262–77.
Panagl, O. (2002), "Vermählen wollte der Magen Sippe dem Mann ohne Minne die
    Maid": Archaisches und Archaisierendes in der Sprache von Wagners *Ring*. In
    U. Müller and O. Panagl (eds), *Ring und Graal*. Würzburg: Königshausen and
    Neumann, 81–91.

Perego, E. (2003), Evidence of Explicitation in Subtitling: Towards a Categorization. *Across Languages and Cultures* 4(1), 63–88.

——(2005), *La traduzione audiovisiva*, Roma: Carocci.

Pérez-González, L. (2009), Audiovisual Translation. In M. Baker and G. Saldahna (eds), *Routledge Encyclopaedia of Translation Studies*, 2nd edn. London: Routledge, 13–20.

Sablich, S. (2002), Tradurre all'epoca dei sopratitoli. *Il Giornale della Musica*, 188.

Stampacchia, E. (2004), *Traduzione e sopratitolaggio. Il caso dell'opera lirica*. Unpublished MA Thesis, University of Pavia.

Telve, S. (1998), Costanti lessicali e semantiche della librettistica verdiana. *Studi di Lessicografia Italiana* 15, 319–47.

Tomaszkiewicz, T. (2009), Linguistic and Semiotic Approaches to Audiovisual Translation. In M. Freddi and M. Pavesi (eds), *Analysing Audiovisual Dialogue. Linguistic and Translational Insights*. Bologna: Clueb, 19–29.

Toury, G. (1995), *Descriptive Translation Studies and Beyond*. Amsterdam: John Benjamins.

Virkkunen, R. (2004), The Source-text of Opera Surtitles. *Meta* 49(1), 89–97.

New York Metropolitan Opera productions

Aida, English titles copyright by Sonya Friedman (1996).

La traviata, English titles copyright by Sonya Friedman (1996).

Luisa Miller, English titles copyright by Sonya Friedman (2001).

EDUARD BARTOLL

The Surtitling in Catalan of Classic Foreign Theatre Plays

This paper focuses on the interlingual electronic surtitling of live classic theatre plays and presents a detailed analysis of the Catalan version of *Macbeth*. Electronic surtitling has been recognized as a professional practice since the 1990s; it is very common in Catalonia and is provided regularly in various Barcelona theatres, such as the Teatre Lliure or the Teatre Nacional de Catalunya and also during theatre festivals, such as Barcelona's Festival Grec or Girona's Temporada Alta. There is a high percentage of classic works, from authors such as William Shakespeare, among the pieces that are surtitled. Apart from the challenges posed by translating such authors, it is important to also consider the differences between drama and theatrical translation, which may not always be apparent.

1. Drama translation as audiovisual translation

One of the debates within audiovisual translation studies is whether drama translation belongs to this area of research. In this regard, Delabastita (1989: 197) suggests that the audiovisual text has much in common with the dramatical text, because of its complexity: "A film constitutes a complex sign, in a way not unlike the theatrical performance sign". However, when considering translation, the author concludes that drama and film present significant semiotic differences because, whilst the structure of a film is pre-determined, in theatre the performance sign is constructed during the performance itself.

But Delabastita does not consider the differences between drama and theatrical text. Espasa (2001: 56), following on from Aragay (1992: 4) and Elam (1980: 3), instead establishes an interesting distinction between the two, "By dramatic text we understand the written text, as having been conceived for the theatre, whilst we use the term theatrical text when the staging in the theatre is being referred to".

Despite the similarities between the translation of dramatic texts and the translation of theatrical texts it is possible to state that, whilst in a dramatic text the images will be created from the written text, in theatrical translation – and in all audiovisual texts – the translation will be determined by the images.

According to Espasa (2001: 28), it is the very question of the creation of images from the written text that produces the paradox of drama translation:

> Starting from a written text, it is necessary to take into account the whole non-verbal dimension of the theatre, but in short the final translated product is another written text, that a theatre company will stage. This paradox contains, in an embryonic form, the recurrent nucleus of the debate about theatrical translation: the uniqueness of theatrical translation, the complex relationship of the text with its non-verbal dimension, and the difficult alliances of the agents of translation with the text and other agents of the theatrical production. (My translation)

Drama translation can be adapted both to the cultural context of the target language during staging and also to the performance of the actors and actresses who speak the target language and use the gestures of the target culture.

Griesel (2000: 26) was probably the first to define this distinction between dramatic translation (*Dramenübersetzung*) and theatrical translation (*Translation im Theater*): "Dramatic translation is a translation fixed in writing that is transmitted to the audience, spoken or sung. It is not a case of a performance in a foreign language, but rather a performance of a translated foreign work" (my translation). Theatrical translation is defined by Griesel (ibid.: 28) as follows:

> Theatrical translation is carried out on a work in a foreign language; the foreign culture is felt and seen and it is necessary to retain the illusion created in the theatre. This field requires new research that goes further than dramatic translation and literary translation, given that in this case extra linguistic factors such as non-verbal communication, and for example gesture or mime, set design or the wardrobe, situational factors and other elements, play an important role. (My translation)

In other words, theatrical translation must be synchronized with the delivery of the source language. For this reason, as stated by Dewolf (2001: 181) when referring to opera surtitles: "The translation cannot be read as an independent text because it forms an integral part of the staging".

Theatre plays can be broadcast live or recorded for cinema, television, video or DVD, among other media; and therefore are also susceptible to translation. Live performances can be translated by means of various methods of AVT, such as simultaneous interpreting, or – the focus of this article – electronic subtitling. In the following subchapters we shall review the process and history of electronic subtitles.

2. Characteristics of electronic subtitling, for both cinema and theatre

Several studies, including those of Gottlieb (1997), Ivarsson (1992), Ivarsson and Carroll (1998), Díaz-Cintas (2001, 2003) and Díaz-Cintas and Remael (2007) provide definitions of electronic subtitling, but in-depth studies on this topic are still rare.

Theatre and opera subtitles are often called surtitles. Actually, surtitles are a type of subtitles characterized by their position on the images in the case of recorded performances, or above the stage in the case of a live performance. In this paper no distinction is made between the two terms, which are used interchangeably, because subtitles can be found in theatre plays or operas, and surtitles in cinemas, especially in festivals. In Spain several companies – including Softitular, Sublimages, Savinen, 36caracteres and Subtitula'm – project subtitles using this electronic system.

Before focussing on the subtitling of plays, it may be useful to review the basic characteristics of general subtitling in order to gain a better understanding of this practice.

Film subtitles projected in cinemas or broadcast on television, consist of a maximum of 30 to 40 characters per line, and do not normally exceed two lines. A subtitle should not last more than six seconds or less than one, even if it consists of a very short word. Generally, subtitles last between two and four seconds. In opera subtitling the six seconds duration is frequently exceeded.

In principle, the maximum number of characters per subtitle is similar for cinema, theatre and opera; however, theatre and opera subtitles may at times have more space available. In the Gran Teatre del Liceu the surtitles often occupy up to three lines, and during the English language production of *Bollywood The Show*, staged at the Tívoli theatre in Barcelona in 2008, with subtitles in Spanish, the subtitle screen consisted of seven lines of twenty-six characters per line, although it should be noted that speech was scarce and slow.

Subtitling, of course, involves the transformation of an oral text into a written text. This shift creates additional challenges for the translator, who must contend with time and space constraints and also reconstruct the fluidity of orality within the usually more rigid structure of the written language.

Another challenge of subtitling is frequently referred to as "translator vulnerability" (Díaz-Cintas 2003: 43–7): the translator may feel "exposed" in front of an audience who have immediate access to both the original and the translation. This perception of vulnerability affects the decision making process behind many translation solutions and may be a major inconvenience for the translator especially when translating classical texts, due to audience expectations.

3. The process of creating subtitles

Before subtitling a film or a theatre play, it is necessary to spot the text. This task is carried out by the spotter, who must mark the entrance and the exit points of the subtitles and therefore determine appropriate time units. According to Ivarsson (1992: 87):

> One of the most important features of a subtitler's work is timing, a process whereby a reasonable balance is struck between the rhythm, the phrases and the logical divisions of the dialogue and appropriate time units and line lengths for the subtitles he is planning to write.

Correct spotting is important, as it is much easier for the audience to understand what is happening and what is said if the lines of text correspond to the discourse on screen or stage. Ideally, the translator should undertake the spotting process, but even with theatre plays this is not always the case. Ivarsson (ibid.: 153) warns that, "The fact that the final titles are not cued by the translator but by a technician may aggravate the inadequacy of the subtitling".

In the case of theatre subtitles it is necessary to have a recent recording of the staging in order to determine timing and duration of the subtitles. Unfortunately, theatre companies do not always understand this requirement and sometimes only provide an audio recording of the show. Clearly, visual elements are vital in order to understand the play, adopt suitable translation strategies and produce adequate subtitles.

Once the subtitles have been created, they are recorded with the audiovisual text. The electronic subtitles are saved in an electronic file, which is then projected by means of a special software program at the same time as the film or play in a LED backlit screen, with orange or red letters and several typographic limitations. In the case of theatre and opera, the screen is usually situated above the stage. Theatre subtitles can be also produced in PowerPoint format and projected as slides. Some opera theatres now have small liquid crystal screens on seat backs, which, as well as providing the option of activating subtitles, also allow spectators to choose their preferred language. In Barcelona's Gran Teatre del Liceu, for example, this system was introduced in 2001 and provides translations in Catalan, Spanish and English.

In the case of a film, projection of the subtitles can be done automatically with a system based on timecodes. Manually projected electronic subtitles tend to be found in live performances. Again, ideally the projection should be handled by the translator. In theatre and opera this is a must, since the rhythm of the production may vary from day to day and an actor might skip a fragment or change the order of some elements of speech.

Audiences are relatively unaware of this process, and frequently ask if the translator writes subtitles during the production. Whilst this is not surprising, it is disconcerting that some theatre companies themselves frequently underestimate the translator's role. Many directors view the presence of subtitles as an inconvenience and they often ensure that the screen for subtitles is placed far from the stage, causing reading difficulties for the audience.

Often, during dress rehearsals there is no regard for the translator's need to check the rhythm of the production, in order to see whether the subtitles enter and exit when required or whether the positioning of information corresponds to the actions of the actors. Dress rehearsals are usually organized to check the text or the positioning of the actors on the stage and is rarely done at the actual rhythm of the production. To render the translator's work even more difficult, during the performance s/he frequently must sit in a corner of the theatre with an incomplete view of the stage.

4. The history of electronic subtitling

Electronic subtitling was created in 1984 by a Florentine architect, Fabrizio Fiumi, who registered it under the trademark of Softitler, as Fiumi himself declared in an interview for the Montreal paper *Le Devoir* on 18 August 1990. The invention was brought about by a fascination for audiovisual media, especially for the cinema, awakened in him during a stay in Canada and the United States. The following year, from 12 to 16 December, the system was launched at the Florence Independent Cinema Festival. Further reasons for this invention include the requirement to reduce the costs of film subtitling and the desire to provide subtitles without burning them upon the image.

Opera surtitles were first shown in 1983 with the opera *Elektra* by Richard Strauss, which was performed at the Hummingbird Centre in Toronto, at the time called the O'Keefe. Linde (1967) quoted and translated by Ivarsson and Carroll (1998: 19), was an early proponent of the subtitling of plays:

> Since it is too much to expect the audience to know the language well enough to understand the text, a bank of lights should be placed above the stage displaying, in the manner of outdoor electric displays for advertising slogans and news flashes, a continuous [...] translation.

Regarding subtitles for theatre and opera, Gambier (2003: 176) states that: "No research has yet been carried out on the different expectations of opera lovers and novices when they read subtitles". But, later on the same page, it is stated that "in an audience poll, approximately 80 per cent gave their approval". In fact, Sario and Oksanen (1996: 195–6) argue that whilst theatre and opera directors feel that surtitles can be distracting and result in an impoverishment of the artistic sentiment of the play, audiences like them:

> The ordinary audience has accepted surtitling very well. According to several surveys carried out in France between 1987 and 1992, nearly 96% of the individuals asked had a positive opinion about the surtitles, in Paris as well as in Marseille, Toulon, Lyon, Angers, Lille ... (My translation)

A concrete example of surtitling into Catalan of the staging of the classic theatre play *Macbeth*, by William Shakespeare, and a comparison with the staging text and drama translation, will allow us to observe the differences between drama translation and theatrical translation.

5. *Macbeth* by Cheek by Jowl

The play analysed here is a staging of *Macbeth* by the Cheek by Jowl Company, directed by Declan Donnellan, with set design by Nick Ormerod. The production was staged at the Teatre de Salt in Girona, during the Festival Temporada Alta, from the 1st to the 4th October 2009 and is a coproduction by Cheek by Jowl, barbicanbite10, Les Gémeaux/Sceaux/Scène Nationale, the Koninklijke Schouwburg in the Hague, the Grand Théâtre in Luxembourg, the Théâtre du Nord in Lille and the Centre Dramatique du Théâtre in Namur.

Cheek by Jowl was founded in 1981 by Declan Donnellan and Nick Ormerod. The founding manifesto sets out the company's dedication to re-examining classic texts, avoiding mises-en-scène and conceptual set designs, in order to emphasize the actor's work. Cheek by Jowl have presented 10 previously unseen classic European texts in England, among them *Le Cid* by Corneille and *Andromaque* by Racine. By 2008, they had also brought some 13 works of Shakespeare to the stage.

Macbeth is the great tragedy of fiction. A man and a woman, united by ambition, are destroyed in the midst of a terrible blood bath. Shakespeare wrote *Macbeth* during his mature phase, after *King Lear* and before *Coriolanus*, between 1505 and 1506. The work is often considered to be a study of human ambition, embodied in Macbeth and his wife. However a reading centred on the presence of the witches and on their interactions with the protagonist, along with the traits and actions of other characters, would suggest that the play is an examination of a central aspect of human nature: evil.

The staging of *Macbeth* by Cheek by Jowl is a new reading of this classic, with a mise-en-scène which conjures up the world of witchcraft, ghosts and prophetic apparitions in an amazing experience of sound and shadows. The tension between Macbeth's character, his acts and his conscience gives Cheek by Jowl's staging a new intensity.

6. Comparison between the English staging text, the Catalan drama translation and the surtitles

We shall now compare the original with the drama translation and the surtitles – the theatrical translation – in order to identify divergences between the last two. The examples chosen will illustrate the considerable difference between the drama translation and the theatrical one, especially in relation to reduction. In the tables that follow, the first row contains the English original, as presented on stage; the second row shows the Catalan version by Salvador Oliva (2005) and the last row shows the Catalan surtitles.

It should be noted that the English text of the staging diverges from the printed text (*The Complete Works of William Shakespeare*, The Cambridge Text Established by John Dover Wilson for the Cambridge University Press, Chancellor Press, 1990) so the English theatrical text is already different from the the drama one. For example, in Act I, scene II, in the staging by Cheek by Jowl some fragments have been deleted, such as the following part of Duncan's speech:

> He can report,
> As seemeth by his plight, of the revolt
> The newest state.

Part of Malcolm's speech, in the production called Thane, is also missing:

> This is the sergeant,
> Who like a good and hardy soldier fought
> 'Gainst my captivity ... Hail, brave friend!

Let us now proceed to compare the three different versions. Characters' names appear in the staging text as well as in the drama translation, but not in the surtitles, unless these were for the deaf and hard-of-hearing.

Table 6

Example 1	
English staging	MALCOLM What bloody man is that? CAPTAIN Say to the king the knowledge of the broil As thou didst leave it.
Salvador Oliva	DUNCAN Qui és aquest que sagna? (Who is this one who's bleeding?) MALCOLM Digues al rei com estava el combat en el moment que el vas haver d'abandonar. (Say to the king how was the fight the moment you had to leave it)
Surtitles	Qui sagna? Descriu al rei la lluita. (Who's bleeding? Describe the fight to king.)

Note. For Tables 6–18. First row: English original, as presented on stage. Second row: Catalan version by Salvador Oliva (2005). Third row: Catalan surtitles.

In Example 1 in Table 6, Oliva's translation has one hundred characters, whilst the original has ninety. In the surtitle there are only thirty-seven, distributed over two lines. The maximum space available per line is 36 characters, but in this case each person needs a line, since it is a dialogue. The speech in the original lasts six seconds, but the electronic panel only shows the text for five seconds. The reformulation operated in the print translation, which gives a more natural solution in Catalan, is not possible in the surtitle, as the audience obviously must be able to simultaneously read the surtitles and watch the play. This explains the brevity of the surtitle.

Table 7

Example 2	
English staging	CAPTAIN As two spent swimmers, that do cling together And choke their art.
Salvador Oliva	SERGENT les dues parts eren com un parell de nedadors extenuats que, aferrats l'un a l'altre, frenen la seva habilitat. (The two parts were like a pair of exhausted swimmers who, clung together, choke their ability.)
Surtitles	dos nedadors que s'agafen i frenen la seva habilitat. (two swimmers who cling together and choke their ability.)

In Example 2 in Table 7, the surtitle lasts five seconds, which explains the small number of characters. The drama translation, on the other hand, has more than one hundred characters and, more importantly, makes explicit the original comparison "as two spent swimmers" with the addition of the verb *eren com* [were like], which in the surtitles has become a metaphor, since the word *like* is missing.

Table 8

Example 3	
English staging	CAPTAIN The merciless usurper (...) With fortune, on his damned quarrel smiling, Show'd like a rebel's whore.
Salvador Oliva	SERGENT L'implacable Macdonwald (...) i la Fortuna, somrient als seus damnats propòsits se li va comportar com una puta. (The merciless Macdonwald (...) and the Fortune, on his damned quarrel smiling, behaved to him like a whore.)
Surtitles	A l'implacable rebel, la sort li somreia i semblava la seva puta. (To the merciless rebel, the fortune smiled, and looked like his whore.)

In the English staging production, Macdonwald becomes "usurper", whilst
is maintained by Oliva. The surtitle, however, translates "usurper" as *rebel*.
The surtitle also shows paraphrasing, which leads to a much reduced text.
La sort [fortune] becomes the subject of the sentence, and "the merciless
usurper" becomes the recipient.

Table 9

Example 4	
English staging	MACDUFF O horror, horror, horror! Tongue nor heart Cannot conceive nor name thee!
Salvador Oliva	MACDUFF Horror, horror, horror! Ni la llengua ni el cor no tenen noms per poder-te concebre. (Horror, horror, horror! Neither tongue nor heart have names to conceive thee.)

Surtitles	Horror! Ni llengua ni cor et poden concebre o anomenar-te. (Horror! Neither tongue nor heart can conceive thee or mane thee.)

Example 4 in Table 9 shows a common strategy in surtitling, which consists in omitting repeated words, here *horror* (three times) and interjections. Comparing the drama translation with the theatrical one, it can be seen that the definite articles are missing in the surtitle: *ni llengua ni cor* and the verb "name" has been translated literally as *anomenar*. In the drama translation "name" becomes *tenir noms* [to have a name], resulting in a slightly different meaning: "they have no names to conceive thee".

Table 10

Example 5	
English staging	MACBETH What's the matter? MACDUFF Confusion now hath made his masterpiece!
Salvador Oliva	MACBETH i LENNOX Què ha passat? (What has happened?) MACDUFF Ara la destrucció ha fet la seva obra mestra. (Now destruction has made his masterpiece.)
Surtitles	Què ha passat? La confusió ha fet l'obra mestra. (What has happened? Confusion has made the masterpiece.)

In Example 5 in Table 10, there is a shift between the staging text and the drama translation, since "confusion" has become *destrucció* [destruction], but is rendered as *confusió* in the surtitles. The adverb "now" is missing in the theatrical translation, because it can be deduced. The possessive "his" also disappears in the surtitle, which is more natural in Catalan – and shorter – but is rendered in the drama translation.

Table 11

Example 6	
English staging	Most sacrilegious murder hath broke ope The Lord's anointed temple, and stole thence The life o' the building!
Salvador Oliva	El més sacríleg dels assassinats ens ha esberlat el temple de l'ungit del Senyor, i n'ha robat la vida. (The most sacrilegious of murders has broke ope the Lord's anointed temple, and stole its life.)
Surtitles	El més sacríleg dels assassinats ha destruït el temple del Senyor! (The most sacrilegious of murders has destroyed the Lord's temple!)

In Example 6 in Table 11, the theatrical translation is much shorter when compared with both the staging text and the drama translation. The utterance lasts eight seconds, and the actor speaks so fast that there is not enough time for two surtitles. The solution adopted was therefore to have just one surtitle and omit the whole sentence "and stole thence the life o' the building!".

Table 12

Example 7	
English staging	MACDUFF See, and then speak yourselves. Awake, awake!
Salvador Oliva	MACDUFF Contempleu i aleshores ja parlareu vosaltres. Desperteu, desperteu! (Contemplate and then speak yourselves. Awake, awake!)

Surtitles	Mireu, i parleu! Desperteu! (See, and speak! Awake!)

Example 7 is a further instance of reduction. The word "then", which is literally translated in the drama text as *aleshores*, has disappeared in the theatrical translation, since it is quite long, and so has the subject *vosaltres* [you]. Additionally, the repetition of "awake" is only rendered once in the surtitle, which lasts five seconds.

Table 13

Example 8	
English staging	MACDUFF Shake off this downy sleep, death's counterfeit, And look on death itself! up, up, and see The great doom's image!
Salvador Oliva	MACDUFF Traieu-vos del damunt aquest son fluix, gentil imatge de la mort i mireu la mateixa mort. Amunt, amunt! Mireu la imatge del judici! (Shake off this downy sleep, gentil deaht's image, and look at death itself. Up, up! See the doom's image!)
Surtitles	Espolseu-vos el son, imatge de la mort, i mireu-la directament! (Shake off sleep, death's image, and look straight at it!)

In Example 8 in Table 13, the surtitle lasts six seconds, which explains why it is much shorter than both the staging text and the drama translation. Oliva's use of the Catalan phrasal verb *treure's del damunt* [to get somebody/

something off one's back] has been substituted by its synonymous *espol-sar* [shake off], the adjective "downy" has been omitted, and the Catalan *gentil* [gentle], which appears in the drama translation, is missing in the staging text. The final sentence, "the great doom's image", has been omitted in the surtitle.

Table 14

Example 9	
English staging	MACDUFF They were suborn'd: Malcolm and Donalbain, the king's two sons, Are stol'n away and fled; which puts upon them Suspicion of the deed.
Salvador Oliva	MACDUFF Va ser un suborn. Malcolm i Donalbain, els fills del rei, han desaparegut, cosa que fa sospitar d'ells. (It was a bribery. Malcolm and Donalbain, the king's sons, have disappeared, which makes them suspicious.)
Surtitles	Fou un suborn. Els fills del rei han fugit, i són sospitosos. (It was a bribery. The king's sons have fled, and they are suspects.)

Example 9 in Table 14 shows that the passive voice "they were suborn'd" has become a noun both in the drama and theatrical translation: *un suborn* [back translation needed]. In the surtitles, the shorter but more literary form *fou* [was] is used, instead of *va ser*, which is more usual. Both proper names, Malcolm and Donalbain, are omitted in the surtitle and the whole sentence "which puts upon them suspicion of the deed" has become *cosa que fa sospitar d'ells* [which makes (one) suspect them], in the drama translation and *i són sospitosos* [and they are suspects]. The speech lasts seven seconds and is rendered very quickly.

Table 15

Example 10	
English staging	MACBETH We should have else desired your good advice, In this day's council; but we'll take to-morrow. Is't far you ride?
Salvador Oliva	MACBETH Si no, t'hauria demanat l'opinió sobre el Consell d'avui. Ja en parlarem demà. Aniràs lluny? (Otherwise, I would have asked your opinion about today's Council. We'll talk about it tomorrow. Will you go far?)
Surtitles	Volia el teu consell. Demà en parlem. Vas lluny? (I wanted your advise. We will talk about it tomorrow. Are you going far?)

In Example 10 in Table 15 we can observe some major changes between the source and target texts. The long sentence "We should have else desired your good advice in this day's council" has become *Si no, t'hauria demanat l'opinió sobre el Consell d'avui* [Otherwise I would have asked your opinion about today's Council] in the drama translation and *Volia el teu consell* [I wanted your advise] in the theatrical translation. The sentence "Is't far your ride?" has been translated both in the drama and the theatrical translation with the verb *anar* [to go], but in the surtitle the present tense is used, instead of the future, as is the case in the drama translation.

Table 16

Example 11	
English staging	LADY MACBETH Did you send to him, sir? MACBETH I hear it by the way; but I will send: There's not a one of them but in his house I keep a servant fee'd.
Salvador Oliva	LADY MACBETH Li has dit que vingués, senyor? (Did you tell him to come, Sir?) MACBETH Ho he sabut per atzar; però el faré venir. No n'hi ha cap d'aquests que, a casa seva, no tingui algun criat al meu servei. (I've known it by chance; but I will send him to come. There's not a one of them who, in his house, hasn't a servant at my service.)
Surtitles	L'hi has fet arribar? Ho faré, tots tenen criats meus. (Did you send it to him? I will, all of them have servants of mine.)

In Example 11 in Table 16 we find a recurrent strategy in subtitling; that of the use of pronouns. Instead of explicitly rendering the staging sentence "Did you send to him?" as it occurs in the drama translation with *Li has dit que vingués?* [Did you tell him to come?], the surtitle has a combination of two pronouns *l'hi* (Did you send it to him? – referring to the invitation). Since the utterance lasts just six seconds, reduction is required and therefore one sentence is fully omitted, "I hear it by the way". The sentence "they all have servants from me" has been shortened considerably into *tots tenen criats meus* [they all have my servants].

Table 17

Example 12	
English staging	FIRST WITCH Show! SECOND WITCH Show! THIRD WITCH Show! ALL Show his eyes, and grieve his heart; Come like shadows, so depart!
Salvador Oliva	BRUIXA 1 Mostreu-vos. (Show yourselves.) BRUIXA 2 Mostreu-vos. (Show yourselves.) BRUIXA 3 Mostreu-vos. (Show yourselves.) TOTES Mostreu-vos als seus ulls, trenqueu-li el cor, com a ombres que sou, veniu i desapareixeu! (Show yourselves to his eyes, break his heart, like shadows as you are, come and disappear!)
Surtitles	Mostreu! Als seus ulls; ombres marxeu! (Show! To his eyes, shadows depart!)

Example 12 in Table 17 shows the simultaneous speeches of the three witches, which last only eight seconds. There is only one surtitle to replace the whole text, but it should be noted that the theatrical translation also provides a much reduced version of the rhymed sentences:

Show his eyes, and grieve his heart;
Come like shadows, so depart.

Surprisingly, rhyme is not kept in the drama translation, and neither in the surtitle, where the two verses are amalgamated into one sentence.

Table 18

Example 13	
English staging	LADY MACDUFF Wisdom! to leave his wife, to leave his babes, His mansion and his titles in a place From whence himself does fly?
Salvador Oliva	LADY MACDUFF La prudència! Deixar la seva dona i els seus fills, la seva casa i els títols en el lloc d'on fuig? (Prudence! To leave his wife and his children, his house and the titles in the place from whence he flees?)
Surtitles	Savi! Deixar la família, la casa, els títols al lloc d'on fuig? (Wise! To leave the family, the house, the titles in the place from whence he flees?)

In Example 13 in Table 18 the need for reduction leads to considerable syntactical changes in the surtitled text. The noun "wisdom" becomes an adjective, *savi* [wise]; "wife" and "babes" are replaced by the collective noun *família* [family], whilst the possessive adjectives disappear. The whole speech lasts seven seconds and the actress speaks very fast so that creating two surtitles instead of one is not possible.

7. Conclusion

The examples shown here illustrate the wide use of reduction in surtitles. Although such a level of reduction can result in an impoverished target text, it must be remembered that during the staging of a play the original language is retained and the voice and tone of the characters, rhymes, cries, exclamations etc. help the spectator to interpret the play. Indeed, Dewolf (2001: 181) states that in the case of opera: "under-translating is preferable to trying to get every word into titles [as] projected titles are not simply a utilitarian adjunct to understanding but an integral part of the performance and of the creation".

The reduction operated in surtitling often means that source text and theatrical translation can differ considerably. This is of course necessary for a number of reasons such as the rhythm of speech being too fast, characters speaking simultaneously, or technical constraints, such as the distance of the screen from the stage or the space limitations on the screen where the surtitles are projected.

Unfortunately the difficult task of a theatre surtitler is not always fully acknowledged and, as mentioned earlier, s/he may have to endure a lack of cooperation by theatre companies, who frequently regard the surtitler more as a nuisance rather than as a means by which foreign language audiences will be able to better understand their performance.

Further research on theatrical translation should provide interesting insights. In particular, an analysis of the similarities and divergences in the subtitles of a film based on a classic play and the theatre surtitles of a staging of the same text would be particularly interesting.

References

Aragay i Sastre, M. (1992), El llenguatge en la producció teatral de Harold Pinter. Barcelona: Promociones y Publicaciones Universitarias.

Delabastita, D. (1989), Translation and Mass-communication: Film and T.V. Translation as Evidence of Cultural Dynamics. *Babel* 35(4), 193–218.

Dewolf, L. (2001), Surtitling Operas. With Examples of Translations from German into French and Dutch. In Y. Gambier and H. Gottlieb (eds), *(Multi)Media Translation*, Amsterdam: John Benjamins, 179–88.

Díaz-Cintas, J. (2001), *El subtitulado*. Salamanca: Almar.

—— (2003), *Teoría y práctica de la subtitulación, Inglés-Español*, Barcelona: Ariel.

Díaz-Cintas, J. and A. Remael (2007), *Audiovisual Translation: Subtitling*, Manchester: St. Jerome.

Elam, K. (1980), *The Semiotics of Theatre and Drama*. London: Methuen.

Espasa, E. (2001), *La traducció dalt de l'escenari*. Vic: Eumo Editorial.

Gambier, Y. (ed.) (1996), *Les transferts linguistiques dans les médias audiovisuels*. Paris: Presses Universitaires du Septentrion.

—— (2003), Introduction: Screen Transadaptation: Perception and Reception. *The Translator* 9(2), 171–89.

Gottlieb, H. (1997), *Subtitles, Translation & Idioms*. Copenhagen: University of Copenhagen.

Griesel, Y. (2000), *Translation im Theater. Die mündliche und schriftliche Übertragung französischsprachiger Inszenierungen ins Deutsche*. Frankfurt am Main: Peter Lang.

Griesel, Y. (2007), *Die Inszenierung als Translat. Möglichkeiten und Grenzen der Theaterübertitelung*. Berlin: Frank & Timme.

Ivarsson, J. (1992) *Subtitling for the Media: A Handbook of an Art*. Stockholm: Transedit.

Ivarsson, J., and M. Carroll (1998), *Subtitling*. Simrishamn: TransEdit HB.

Linde, E. (1967), *Västöstligt – mest om teater*. Stockholm: Bonniers.

Reed, F. (1990), Le FFM innove avec une méthode révolutionnaire de sous-titrage. *Le Devoir* 18 August.

Sario, M., and S. Oksanen (1996), Le sur-titrage des opéras à l'opéra de Finlande. In Y. Gambier (ed.), *Les transferts linguistiques dans les médias audiovisuels*. Paris: Presses Universitaires du Septentrion, 185–97.

Shakespeare, W. (1990), *The Complete Works of William Shakespeare*. London: Chancellor Press.

—— (2005), *Macbeth*. Translation S. Oliva. Barcelona: Edicions Vicens Vives.

PART TWO

Didactic Applications of Subtitling

CLAUDIA BORGHETTI

Intercultural Learning through Subtitling: The Cultural Studies Approach

1. Introduction

The creation of subtitles has only been seriously employed as a tool for language learning within the past decade. Nonetheless, interest in this recent development in language education research is markedly growing (Williams and Thorne, 2000; Hadzilacos et al., 2004; Talaván Zanón, 2006; Sokoli, 2006). The impulse behind this attention is most likely to be found in the transversal solidarity which has been established between technological development, knowledge acquisition theories, and didactic planning (Calvani, 1998: 44), rather than in the pursuit of diversity within didactic practice. Digitization, the internet, capillary diffusion of technology, and increasingly user-friendly software, far from representing "neutral, static supplements" (ibid., my translation), have actively contributed to changing theoretical and epistemic thought – and consequently didactic thinking – to lead to theories of both knowledge acquisition and teaching that privilege a deliberate construction of knowledge, a meaningful and authentic context for learning, and collaboration (Jonassen, 1994: 37). Like many other professional fields including that of audiovisual translation (AVT) itself, foreign language teaching (FLT) has found in technology[1] both a stimu-

---

1   The renewed consideration given to translation as a means of linguistic acquisition offers one example. The various forms of audiovisual translation, introduced into the foreign language classroom through related technology, have led didactic theory to reconsider the role of translation in language learning, recognizing merits which in the past had been denied (Rogers, 2008).

lus for theoretical renewal and an answer to many of the methodological needs arising in parallel with the assertion of new conceptual principles. This trend is also evident in the extensive affirmation of various forms of network-based language teaching and – more specifically relevant to the topic of this article – in the growing use of intra- or interlingual subtitled videos as language learning tools (Pavesi, 2002; Caimi, 2006).

On a language teaching level, beyond all of the advantages linked to the use of subtitled audiovisual materials (motivational stimulus, visualization of the foreign language and culture, memory power etc.), the active creation of interlingual subtitles offers additional benefits that positively influence language acquisition processes: it engages a broad range of productive abilities such as spelling, writing, and summarizing; it helps develop textual and translation skills; it encourages students to favour more ample semantic and pragmatic reformulation over word-for-word translation in virtue of space and time limitations (Talaván Zanón, 2006: 47); and it lends itself to an additional series of micro-activities such as note-taking, extensive and intensive listening, etc. (Sokoli, 2006). On a didactic level, creating subtitles favours the establishment of constructive learning environments, as it stimulates forms of active learning by introducing realistic and meaningful activities which lead to concrete outcomes (Hadzilacos et al., 2004); it presumes recourse to various codes in order to decipher and comprehend; it encourages metalinguistic reflection, which in turn facilitates strategic thinking and thus learning itself; it frequently necessitates group work and, consequently, forms of "reciprocal teaching" (Palincsar and Brown, 1984) which generally lead to a "community of learner" dynamics (Brown and Campione, 1994).

Within the vast topic of subtitling in foreign language teaching, this article specifically examines the largely unexplored area of audiovisual translation's educational value when used with intercultural aims in the foreign language classroom. Reflection on how this didactic practice can be used to better promote the development of students' cultural and intercultural awareness seems necessary at this time of broad consensus on the idea that foreign language learning must provide the opportunity to approach a foreign culture and, more importantly, to develop intercultural knowledge, attitudes, and skills. Even more significantly, the extent to which the practice of subtitling in foreign language learning corresponds to certain forms of Intercultural Foreign Language Education (IFLE)[2] and, consequently, its intrinsic predisposition for use with intercultural aims is striking. If standard translation already represents a cultural transfer (Katan, 1999), AVT is only made possible through a complex process of reflection and calculation which is intrinsically intercultural. In anticipation of experimental research confirming the thesis here proposed, this article outlines the steps involved in the process of subtitling, isolating and commenting on the principal moments of this process which have a potential educational value in the intercultural sense. This exploratory effort is supported by extensive referencing of the cultural analysis inspired by Cultural Studies, which, after all, has been deeply woven into both translation studies (Bassnett, 2003; Brisset, 2003) and IFLE (Byram, 1988, 1989) for some years now.

Both Intercultural Foreign Language Education (section 1) and Cultural Studies (section 2) are presented in the text that immediately follows, the latter in a manner specifically in line with our aims, given its lengthy history. These brief initial outlines will then permit more efficient concentration on the theoretical and methodological principles that make the creation of interlingual subtitles an opportunity for intercultural acquisition (section 3). They will also facilitate a more effective analysis of the subtitling process from an intercultural educational prospective (section 4).

2. Intercultural Foreign Language Education

This particular form of language teaching, initially established in Europe following studies conducted by Michael Byram in the 1980s, is currently enjoying a remarkable level of international consideration. This fact is

---

2   Intercultural Foreign Language Education is here defined as foreign language teaching whose principal educational goal includes the development of students' intercultural competence (section 1).

evident given the many prestigious European Council publications, to which Byram himself often contributed (Byram and Zarate, 1994; Lázár, 2007), and the number of accomplished scholars from different parts of the world who are currently engaged in the cultural and intercultural dynamics of language teaching.

When Byram began to concentrate on the educational value of linguistic teaching in the early 1980s, the communicative approach was dominant in language education. Inspired by the 1960s notion of "communicative competence", methods based on the communicative approach revolutionized foreign language didactics once and for all, affirming the importance of appropriateness and efficacy in communication alongside linguistic accuracy. Knowledge of a language no longer meant simply mastering its grammatical rules (phonetic, morphological, syntactical etc.) but also acquiring the ability to utilize these rules in a manner appropriate to definite aims, situations, and all the contingent factors related to specific communicative situations. The consequent emphasis on socio-linguistic and pragmatical-linguistic aspects of communication led foreign language teaching to contextualize language for the first time in a wider socio-cultural framework. This cultural turning-point, reached most didactic contexts in the Western world almost contemporaneously and profoundly influenced FLT and still today represents the fundamental basis of "intercultural education discourse".

Nevertheless, if on the one hand foreign culture fully entered into language curricula as a result of communicative methods, often even suggesting both structure and progression by offering "typical situations" and "recurrent linguistic functions"; on the other, for a long period (and often still today) cultural contents were introduced for purely utilitarian purposes, causing the foreign culture presented to students to be fragmentary, anecdotal, and often stereotyped. It was precisely in objection to this notion of the exclusively instrumental value of language and culture that Byram (1998) began to emphasize the profound educational role which linguistic teaching could assume if only it were to tap into the cultural aspects of the languages being studied. In Byram's *Cultural Studies in Foreign Language Education*, published in 1989, his efforts towards an educational renewal of foreign language teaching culminate in the new title designated for the discipline, in which he substitutes "teaching" with "education". Far from representing a terminological afterthought, this change fully corresponds to Byram's comprehensive innovation project, including objectives, contents and methodology.

As regards the ultimate objectives of Foreign Language Education as theorized by Byram, these cannot be defined in terms of readily evident actions (such as, for example, learning to conduct a conversation through means of a foreign code); but rather they reside in the development of cognitive observational skills and a critical analysis of cultural factors, as well as in the maturation of intellectual and emotional attitudes such as the suspension of judgment or openness to diversity. Beyond this, while students practice understanding the cultural system of which the foreign language they study is an integral part and they become aware of the pervasiveness of cultural factors, they are also stimulated and guided in examining their own cultures in an objective and analytical manner (Kramsch, 1993, 1998). In short, it can be stated that the aims of intercultural learning revolve around an overarching educational goal, that of intercultural competence (IC). Even within the seemingly interminable array of definitions attributed to IC (Deardorff, 2006: 242), an individual possessing a good level of IC can be defined as "someone who has a critical or analytical understanding of (part of) their own and other cultures – someone who is conscious of their own perspective, of the way in which their thinking is culturally determined, rather than believing that their understanding and perspective is natural" (Byram 2000: online).

In parallel with these objectives, the main content that IFLE students must acquire beyond the linguistic code *per se*, is a method of observation and cultural inquiry equally applicable to both the foreign culture and their own culture. This is essentially the comparative method of the ethnographer, which is a method of observing and relating a base culture to a foreign culture, and represents a tool that deters ethnocentrism and encourages a conception of the strange as familiar and the familiar as strange.

Finally, as regards methodology, this partly coincides with content, since these two factors coexist within an exemplary use in teaching of the same comparative method that the student is meant to acquire, while it is further enriched through specific attention being given to the personal motivations and experiences of the students (Byram, 1989: 18–20).

Notions such as "intercultural speaker" (Byram and Zarate, 1994; Kramsch, 1998), "intercultural (communicative) competence" (Byram, 1997), and "tertiary socialization" (Byram, 1989) or "third place" (Kramsch, 1993), have served to formalize the new theoretical language of the intercultural approach, based largely on anthropology and social psychology. This terminology soon found a didactic correspondence in precise educational goals and evaluation criteria, as well as in a number of methodological solutions.

Many theoretical arguments which have formulated and contributed to establishing IFLE in the past twenty years can also support renewed discourse on "intercultural citizenship education".[3] Necessitated by unprecedented educational challenges caused by phenomena which (language) teachers have been facing over the past few years such as globalization and internationalization, reflections of this nature represent the immediate continuation of the intercultural approach, where the purpose of foreign language teaching and "the duty of teachers, [is] not only to combine utility and educational value, but also to show learners how they can and should engage with the international globalized world in which they participate" (Byram, 2008: 229).

3. Cultural Studies for Intercultural Foreign Language Education

When Byram (1989) foresaw the possibility for a broader horizon of ultimate educational objectives concerning the foreign language teaching of his time, Cultural Studies was the first field of study to which he turned.

3   Before being conducted on a "worldwide", "global", or, indeed, "intercultural" scale
     (Guilherme, 2002; Byram, 2008), discussion on citizenship education within IFLE
     had already sparked some interest in relation to the concept of European citizenship
     (Byram, 1996).

Once he had identified the privileged access to an educational dimension that the link between language and culture offered, he considered it necessary to explore the field which, among the entire range of human and social sciences, most closely examined cultural products as tools for understanding everyday social, political, and cultural practice. What is interesting to note, however, is that Byram's use of the term "Cultural Studies", refers only in part to the school of thought that has been dedicated to the systematic study of culture since the end of the 1950s, first prevalently in Great Britain and then in a good part of the world.[4] He prefers, in fact, to use the expression "Cultural Studies" in generic terms, "provided it is taken to refer to all aspects of culture as a way of life, to include all those dimensions which an anthropological ethnography, a history of art, crafts and literature and contemporary social and political history would describe" (1988: 17).

Nonetheless, Cultural Studies taken specifically to mean the original school of thought itself, can also offer an enormous contribution to the creation of intercultural methodologies – including those based on the creation of subtitles specifically – precisely thanks to those aspects which, starting from the conceptualization of its topic of study, have determined its absolute originality within cultural theory in the 1960s.

Cultural Studies is thus the study of culture. Far from representing a banality, the issue of defining just what is meant by "culture" perfectly exemplifies the atmosphere in which Cultural Studies was formed. It was the response to this dispute that both constituted the creation of this field of study itself, and offered the most famous contribution of Cultural Studies to the history of thought in the twentieth century. For Cultural Studies, "culture" is:

> a set of transactions, processes, mutations, practices, technologies, institutions, out of which things and events (such as movies, poems or world wrestling bouts) are produced, to be experienced, lived out and given meaning and value to in different

---

4   For reasons of space limitation, it would be impossible to do justice to the intense history of Cultural Studies here. However, a long bibliography of material is available for consultation on the topic, which includes the work of Lutter and Reisenleitner (2002) and During (2005).

ways within the unsystematic network of differences and mutations from which they emerged to start with (During, 2005: 6).

Culture thus does not end at artistic expression or the moral teachings of individual geniuses called upon to educate and save the masses. Quite the contrary, it is the masses who, from the end of the Second World War, found representational (and at times expressive) means within the so-called category of "mass popular culture", no longer regarded as a menace to "culture" but rather as one of its integral – and even productive – factors.

It is clear how an idea of culture such as that diffused by Cultural Studies could prove decisive for IFLE: both the production of so-called "high culture" and phenomena typical to everyday life (gestures, habits, objects) of the foreign country can be placed in relation with one another and can even help to better describe and explain each other. What renders Cultural Studies decisive for intercultural linguistic education, however, is its reconstruction of culture through the pluralism of texts[5] which together constitute and represent it. A text becomes an opportunity to ask: "Who [is speaking]? When and where? With or to whom? Under what institutional or historical constraints?" (Clifford, 1986: 13). It is thus witness to the social reality that is evolving and transforming above and beyond the process of codification that led to the creation of a particular television programme, painting, or specific social event; the text reveals something about the ontological truth, the socio-cultural context, and the underlying epistemological operation that the product in part hides and disguises, and in part lets us catch a glimpse. Extremely interesting both from educational and translational standpoints, the text is also a constant self-reflection on the cultural presumptions and conditioning that influences the process of its interpretation: No process of interpretation is value-free, just as no

---

5   The term "text" is intended in its acceptation within Cultural Studies: "text is a metaphor that invokes the constitution of meaning through the organization of signs into representations. [...] Since images, sounds, objects and practices are sign systems which signify with the same fundamental mechanism as a language we may refer to them as cultural texts. Hence, dress, television programmes, images, sporting events, pop stars etc. can all be read as texts" (Barker, 2004: 199).

description can be objective. As a consequence, individuals who carry out these operations (in our case the student/audiovisual translator) must be aware of the multiple levels of conditioning that accompany them in their manipulation of the text.

4. Creation of subtitles for intercultural education purposes

The creation of subtitles is a complex activity and requires time and patience: the student must acquire confidence with the means, comprehend the verbal message and put it into relation with information carried by non-verbal codes, choose the most suitable translation strategies, then proceed to reduction and synchronization etc. As we will see in this paragraph as well as in the next, this complexity constitutes an opportunity to stimulate the intercultural acquisition process, since, given the quality of the operations which must be undertaken, it first induces inquiry, doubt, and modesty, and then requires definitive decision-making, thus fostering responsibility. Following is a list of those theoretical and methodological principles inspired by IFLE and Cultural Studies (sections 1 and 2) that seem to make the most of such complexity for the development of students' intercultural competence.

4.1. Authentic task in simulation

As emphasized in literature (Hadzilacos et al., 2004: 680; Talaván Zanón, 2006: 49), the authenticity of the assigned task represents one of the strong points of didactic methodologies which concentrate on the creation of subtitles. The students, like professional audiovisual translators, subtitle scenes from a film, a commercial, or part of a TV programme, and in doing so they exploit and develop their communicative-linguistic competencies in the foreign language, at times without even being aware of this.

From an intercultural perspective, however, the authentic nature of this task plays an even more important role. Since IC acquisition is a complex process involving both cognitive and affective factors, it is necessary to utilize dynamics which comprehensively involve students. One way of achieving this is to make students immediately aware of relationship networks that underlie subtitling, beginning with those in which they themselves become protagonists as they subtitle (for example, the relationship between director and subtitler, or that between subtitler and the target audience.) In this way, as we shall see (section 3.4.), it is possible to make students aware of the importance of the assignment. Subtitling then becomes an even more authentic act, as it is contextualized within the complex socio-professional framework in which it is usually undertaken. Making students aware of this also involves asking them to take simulation to its extreme, where they participate pretending to be a team of professionals. In order to make the translator's social function (and, consequently, the responsibility assumed) more visible and deeply felt, it is possible to frame the subtitling activity in a context of "community service": students are instructed to subtitle a film produced by the culture whose language they are studying for the use of their peers in other classes who do not speak the language. In this way, not only do the students assume the role of "experts" in that specific languaculture, but they themselves experience the responsibility of those who translate from one language and culture to another.

In intercultural education, also, students' full awareness of the didactic process in terms of expected results and strategies used to reach these results is an integral part of authenticity. While in the case of mere linguistic acquisition the role given to meta-cognition can be marginal or come into play only at the monitoring level (Krashen, 1985), in intercultural-linguistic acquisition, awareness and comprehension of the educational process, along with the individual's self-monitoring of his own learning progress, are fundamental (Borghetti, 2008: 210–11). This not only means that it is necessary to make students fully aware of the linguistic-intercultural objectives of the subtitling activity, but it assumes that the instructor must accompany them throughout the process, continuously encouraging them to reflect on the source text (ST) culture and the target text (TT) culture, at levels of both verbal and non-verbal discourse, as well as at a more general cultural level.

4.2. *Interlingual subtitles*

The types of subtitles most appropriate for activities aimed at fostering intercultural learning beyond linguistic skills are interlingual, because unlike intralingual subtitles, these involve two languages and two cultures. With interlingual subtitles, students are first external spectators of the video produced in the source language and culture, and mainly work to decode the text according to their own cultural schemata. During the second phase, however, they move from representing a simple (foreign) audience to becoming translators. At this point they must leave behind their original guise, and, with the help of the available tools (the assistance of teachers and peers, internet, electronic dictionaries, other videos etc.), they must examine the video document and the culture it represents through both internal and estranged lens. This process, again, a decoding one, is rooted in interpretive axioms as far as possible in line with those of the source audience, and announces the last, delicate phase of encoding for the target audience. Here the student must make translational choices which "help the target audience to locate the film so firmly in the original contextual conditions that they will not consider interpreting the signs in terms of their own culture", considering that they "should have viewing conditions, as well as a basis for interpretation, comparable to those of the original audience" (Niemeier, 1991: 152).

Taking all of this into account, it becomes clear how intralingual subtitles are not equally suitable for aims of an intercultural nature, seeing as they exclude the dialogue, mediated by the student/translator, between the two languacultures involved in interlingual subtitling. A different position still must be taken about reversed subtitling: if the video is in the student's languaculture, who must subtitle in a foreign language, the greatest risk is a lack of estrangement, since the video will immediately make factors that are very unclear to the target audience appear natural and culturally neutral to the student. Having said this, it is possible to adapt reverse subtitling, if one is careful to propose this activity to classes who already have a good level of intercultural awareness, regardless of their linguistic level.

4.3. Video as cultural text

Screen translation, in general, has the merit of rendering the translation process less immediate and linear than traditional translation for students. Regarding subtitling, this is due either to the necessity of simplifying and omitting small parts of dialogue because of technical constraints of space and time for example, or because of synchronization requirements. At any rate, in acquiring experience of these factors, students must stop and question the text as a cultural product, rather than conceiving it as a sequence of signs to translate (Olk, 2002). First and foremost, students can easily experience the video as a complex entity once they realize that the meaning of the verbal exchange to be translated is strongly influenced by information transmitted through other semiotic systems such as non-verbal communication (paralanguage, kinesics, proxemics, chronemics etc.), music, sound, images, camera movements etc. Revealing the intense interweaving which constitutes all text typologies, this multi-modality adopts a fundamental role. Discovery of this complexity by students is a precursor to that of the depth of the text, in the way of Cultural Studies. While a text presents itself as an autonomous reality with an end in itself, it masks cultural belief, value and customs systems that may occasionally profoundly influence an audience's reading of settings, situations or the words spoken. If this depth is of primary interest to the professional subtitler, who must bear in mind implicit cultural messages in order to also make verbal messages understandable to outsiders, it is also of keen interest in education, where reaching a "thick description" (Geertz, 1973) through cultural awareness and analysis constitutes one of the first intercultural objectives.[6]

---

6   For a few examples of reviews of the objectives linked to intercultural development, see Byram (1997: 57–64) and Borghetti (2008: 289–98).

4.4. Student/subtitler's multiple responsibilities

Many of the objectives linked to the acquisition of intercultural competence (for example ability to observe and listen, mediation, assertiveness, and decision making etc.) can be attained by focusing on the multiple responsibilities that translators (audiovisual or otherwise) face, since, "beyond languages, translation establishes relationships among people" (Brisset, 2003: 101). Translators must indeed manipulate the text keeping in mind the "multiple divided loyalties" (Pym, 2010: 172–3) which link them to the figures involved in every translation process: first of all, the author, the ST, the ST culture and the target audience (besides the client and the publisher, who, however, do not have equivalents in didactic simulation and therefore can be placed aside for our purposes here).

Respecting the author and the ST, in the specific case of subtitling, not only entails avoiding distortion of textual form and content but also operating in such a way that subtitles do not impede viewing of the video (for example by monopolizing the viewer's attention due to excessive length, altering the rhythm and tone of the dialogues, flattening speech or socio-linguistic variables of the language etc.).

The responsibility that students/subtitlers must perceive regarding the source culture is even more delicate, because their choices, and more specifically "the type of strategy used will impact on TC perception of the SC – preserving 'local colour', perpetuating (positive or negative) stereotypes, undermining or highlighting cultural specificities, possibly even creating cross-cultural misunderstanding" (Ramière, 2006: 156–7). The translators' function thus assumes notable ethical tones, and forces them to reflect on their own role as mediators between one culture and another. Among the possible reactions to this responsibility is recourse to foreignization strategies which, underlining the peculiarity of the foreign culture, have the benefit of reducing the risk of ideological dominance of the target culture (Venuti, 1995). This approach also, undoubtedly, has the advantage of drawing on the students' linguistic creativity. In an educational context, and especially with beginner classes, it would seem more appropriate to adopt a humble approach (Izzo, 1970), which, without exalting faithfulness to the text, would help emphasize the importance of

respect for the audiovisual material and the source languaculture; in the
end, the students are simply learning to observe, penetrate and understand
the ST culture. This appears even more sensible if one considers that more
cautious criteria pertaining to approaching the text do not at all exclude
the adoption of opportune foreignization strategies such as retention/
borrowing or calque.

Yet another factor to which students must constantly pay attention
is the target audience – the receiver of and, in the end the motive itself
for, their subtitling efforts. At first glance, this relationship appears less
complex than the one which links the students to the source audience. In
general language students are, in fact, part of the cultural group for which
they are translating, and this, if we momentarily exclude the constraints
of subtitling, should make cultural-linguistic subtitling choices rather
easy, since the students should know or at least be able to imagine which
among the cultural references or implicits would not be received without
a mediation through themselves. This immediacy risks are theoretical only,
however, given that students are not always sufficiently familiar with cultural items belonging to their own wider cultural context. Beyond this,
even if the task were to prove easy, this ease should not pass unobserved
by the class: if this relationship appears simpler than those previously
discussed, it is due to a shared cultural knowledge which makes everything seem more fluid and natural, present in the case of the TT culture
but mostly absent in the case of the ST culture. Furthermore, this does
not lessen the translator's responsibility to his audience: students must
never forget that they are offering a linguistic-cultural mediation without
which the receiver would have no access to the text, and therefore those
who read their subtitles trust their work and mediation. Regarding the
unique characteristics of subtitling, students must be very aware that if a
reduction of the language of the original script is inevitable,[7] this can be
risky on an intercultural level since it raises the level of the directness of

7   Subtitling tends to condense the original dialogue by 20–40%, partly as a result
     of the "diasemiotic" process of transcodification, and "partly due to technical and
     perceptional constraints" (Gottlieb, 2004: 87).

pragmatic features. As has emerged from recent research conducted by Pinto (2010: 273), this can have as a consequence an effect of unintended impoliteness, especially on audiences who are unfamiliar with the ST culture and who, due to complete ignorance of the language, are forced to focus their attention on the subtitled text, "which implies less attention to paralinguistic and visual cues".

4.5. Subtitling as interpretation

The multiple responsibilities of the students/subtitlers, for reasons already mentioned, lead them to assume "a meta-perceptual position" (Katan, 2009: 297), to occupy, according to Kramsch (1993), a "third place" with respect to those of the ST and TT cultures. However, this overarching role must not allow students to forget that their mediation is in no way neutral, just as the translator/subtitler is never transparent (Venuti, 1995). On the contrary, from a semiotic point of view, the individual who translates/ subtitles "occupies the same position as the spectators of the original film version. Consequently it is not a 'firsthand' interpretant the translator is generating" (Niemeier, 1991: 150), but rather one already conditioned by contextual and personal factors. The invitation to self-reflection deriving from Cultural Studies should work to caution students to consult with peers and their teacher when subtitling, not only from a strictly linguistic point of view, but also as far as their personal interpretation of the text is concerned. Even when dealing with relatively straightforward audiovisual sequences that do not present particular problems of polysemy, it must be stressed that every reading, including that of the translator, is cultural and thus conditioned.

5. The subtitling process in an intercultural perspective

This section, dedicated to commenting on the subtitling process as a progression of didactic actions aimed at fostering better intercultural education, presents a number of methodological solutions that allow this process to be carried out contextually and in parallel with linguistic-communicative objectives.

Audiovisual subtitling progression is here articulated in five steps, which indubitably contain "the most elementary pragmatic distinction that one can specify as an 'act of translation', that is to say, the stages of reading, drafting and revision" (Morini, 2007: 100, my translation). The process has been kept purposefully broad, in line with both the exploratory objectives of this article and the reality of the subtitling progression itself, in which an overlapping of stages is much more prominent than their clear sequential distinction. The articulation of these steps as they are proposed herein is primarily informed by IFLE (Borghetti, 2008: 102), Audiovisual Translation (Bartrina and Espasa, 2005: 94–7), and various studies dedicated to the creation of subtitles for the purpose of foreign language learning (Williams and Thorne, 2000: 219–21; Neves, 2004: 131–7; McLoughlin and Lertola, forthcoming).

5.1. Presentation and motivation

This first step is of fundamental importance in language education and fulfils two distinct but integrated needs. On the one hand, the need to increase students' awareness of the didactic process, so that they can recall related knowledge already acquired in order to better contextualize the new knowledge they are about to access; on the other, the need to direct students towards a mindset that better fosters learning on an emotional level, for example by stimulating their curiosity and minimizing any fear they might have due to the novelty of the proposed activity.

For our purposes, presentation of the activity above all entails exposing its linguistic and intercultural objectives to the students, before introducing them to the theoretical and technical aspects of subtitling, and
allowing them to become familiar with the video materials that they will
be using.[8]

A brief frontal explanation elucidating the choice of subtitling in pursuit of intercultural objectives in all likelihood will prove the most effective
method for exposing the activity's didactic aims. This explanation must
clarify what the desired intercultural objectives are by introducing some
key concepts related to intercultural competence and audiovisual texts. A
direct approach is also preferable in order to favour a relationship of trust
between the teacher and students, especially considering that in the initial
stages most of all, the students will have to allow themselves be guided
through complex and completely new didactic experiences.

A wide variety of activities can be used to introduce the audiovisual
material, along with subtitling itself, to stimulate student motivation:
brainstorming on the video and the genre to which it belongs; surfing the
internet to find useful and/or curious information about the director or
the actors; small tasks aimed at familiarizing students with subtitling software etc. To ensure that this first phase begins to guide students toward
adopting a mentality of critical analysis and helps them to develop their
awareness of the means to be employed, it could be useful to show part

---

8   It is possible to utilize a wide range of filmed materials: movies, documentaries,
     advertisements, soap operas, etc. Solely for reasons of convenience, rather than due
     to any difference in educational value, this article exclusively refers to the subtitling
     of films. What is of cardinal importance, however, is the choice of materials to be
     used: ideal filmed material would be represented by a multi-layered cultural prod-
     uct, in which cultural elements that are relatively simple to decode, even for the
     foreign viewer (the setting and characters, for example), are accompanied by other
     more difficult elements such as situational conventions (behaviour during specific
     events, for example), implicit cultural factors (wisecracks, omissions made on the
     conversational level, etc.), socio-linguistic variables (accent, register, etc.), and so on.
     Another desirable level of analysis would be that of the format and the genre of the
     filmed material chosen, which, especially in the case of film genres, often contain
     traces of the stylistic traditions from which the product stems.

of a film with interlingual subtitles, whose original language is the students' native language. In this way students can practice critical thinking by commenting on the choices made by the subtitler, but also attempt to "correct" his/her work, thus directly familiarizing themselves with the fact that different translational solutions always exist. Another possible introductory activity could consist in active participation in intralingual subtitling: students subtitle a few seconds of a video of their choice in their own language. By completing this task, they will reach an awareness of some of the limits imposed by subtitling (those of space and time, but also, quite possibly, those linked to the passage from oral to written codes). Beyond this, students will be able to experience the challenge of choosing just one translational option.

5.2. Viewing

Even though students will only subtitle a brief film clip,[9] it is important for them to watch the entire film at this second stage, so that they have an overview of the cultural product with which they have been presented. For reasons of time limitation, especially when working with beginner or intermediate classes, it is possible to utilize the subtitles already supplied on the DVD (either intralingual or interlingual, at the teacher's discretion). This, of course, with the exception of those sequences that have been chosen for the subtitling activity, since all linguistic and (inter)cultural activity will be concentrated on those excerpts later.

At the language educational level, this stage can be described as dedicated to a global approach to the text, in which the goal of developing students' listening skills is pursued by assisting them in using all-encompassing comprehension strategies which involve utilizing both their encyclopedic knowledge and decoding skills which go beyond the verbal. Either

9   Considering, for example, a total didactic commitment of ten hours entirely dedicated to subtitling, the film clip to be subtitled should not be longer than four to five minutes.

individually or in groups, students will watch their assigned clip repeatedly, before verifying their hypotheses of comprehension against a copy of the script.

It is at this stage, conducted via a global approach that exploration of the source video's culture begins. The notion of "comprehension" thus extends to include the cultural level, through formulating questions and hypotheses about the film, the ST audience, ST culture and ST language, and, consequently, about the students' own culture(s). At this point students should not in any way think they have reached definitive responses, as these would risk being hurried and highly influenced by stereotypes. It is the teacher's responsibility to ensure that this does not happen, and if it seems that students are too confident with the swift answers they have supplied themselves, the teacher can move on to the next phase earlier than planned (section 4.3.), so that this stage of observation coincides as far as possible with the following phase of research.

As the translator, the student/subtitler must reflect on various questions. Firstly, regarding the text: "What kind of text is the original? Must the newly created text belong to the same textual variety?" (Morini, 2007: 104, my translation). Then regarding the audience: What audience represents the film's "model reader"? (Eco, 2004). Who will be the receiver of the subtitled version? Students must also reflect on the ST culture: Are there settings, phenomena or situations in the sequence to be subtitled that can or cannot be found in the TT culture? If not, why is this so? Is it possible to find a functional equivalent in the TT culture of this specific phenomenon? Finally, students must consider one last series of questions concerning the language of the clip: What variety of language are the characters speaking (on diatopic, diastratic, and diaphasic levels especially)? Are there any expressions that are unclear? Are there any hidden cultural meanings? Are there strange gestures or facial expressions whose meaning is unclear?

On a methodological level, this phase can be carried out using various activities, which can range from highly structured (such as handing out analytical worksheets prepared by the teacher as group work), to freer procedures (such as brainstorming, web diagrams focused on key expressions such as "the film", "the audience", "the language of the characters"), or similar worksheets created by the students themselves. The choice of activities to be carried out, just as that of the language used to give instructions, is left up to the teacher to decide, on the basis of class level, time available and the specific details relative to the chosen filmed material.

5.3. Research

In the second stage, with the progressive shift in focus from the textual to the linguistic level, video analysis becomes more and more detailed and minute. In this third stage, the study proceeds, accompanied by research conducted on the internet, dictionaries, text corpora, and, if necessary, questions posed to natives of the ST culture. This activity has multiple aims: to verify, if possible, assumptions formulated earlier (section 4.2.) by collecting information on the genre of the film to be subtitled, the cultural features identified, the ST language variety and other non-verbal factors; to conduct research on the TT culture; to acquire new, more detailed information on the film, the director, etc.; to identify conventional factors related to style and subtitling choices in the TT language etc., by learning more about films of the same genre, especially when the clip to be subtitled belongs to a highly formulaic film genre (such as westerns, wacky comedies, horror films). It is important that students make notes on all information gathered in a journal, which can either be individual or collective, so that this information does not end up lost or forgotten. They can also write any questions in their journals which remain unanswered (expressions which have not been sufficiently decoded), as well as their first attempts at translation etc.

Beyond these objectives, this third phase contains a highly educational component, as on the one hand it leads to humility through having to reconsider initial assumptions, while on the other it stimulates curiosity and openness towards the foreign culture. Consequently, in addition to reinforcing certain components necessary for intercultural competence such as the acquisition of "knowledge" and "skills", these research activities can also influence students' "attitudes". Not only do students have the opportunity to develop the "ability to acquire new cultural knowledge and cultural practices [and] to interpret a document or event from another culture, to explain it and relate it to documents or events from one's own" (Byram, 1997: 57), but they are also impelled to act on their "curiosity and openness, readiness to suspend disbelief about other cultures and belief about [their] own" (ibid.: 61).

This procedure should be intended, as shown here, as the third step in the subtitling process solely for purposes of convention, and should rather be presented to students as a resource which can guide them throughout the entire process of appropriate subtitling, and – even more importantly – as an effective process of linguistic and cultural knowledge acquisition. On this basis, web-based activities to be completed as group work recommended at this stage can also be proposed to the class prior to and after this point.

5.4. Timing and translating

This fourth stage, which in literature is often broken down into two sub-stages (Neves, 2004: 134–7; Bartrina and Espasa, 2005: 94–6), is mainly dedicated to technically and linguistically oriented tasks, so that students, preferably in groupwork, can undertake the actual subtitling of the assigned film clip. At the same time, this step will have been enriched by the research and reflection carried out previously, both in terms of new knowledge acquired (and recorded) and in terms of a more solid level of relevant linguistic-cultural awareness. Once relevant cultural themes have been identified, discussed, and analyzed, the linguistic-translational task, rather than representing the final objective of the exercise and the only learning effort, is more easily contextualized in a vision of the language as one of many tangible demonstrations of culture, thus leading to a privileged access to its comprehension (Borghetti, 2008: 103).

Leaving aside all detail regarding the technical procedures of subtitling, for which McLoughlin and Lertola (in this publication) in particular are recommended as references, what is of interest here are the effects the process of recoding has on the acquisition of intercultural competence, when preceded by an intense decoding process.

After identifying and analysing the most culturally indicative verbal exchanges in a well-chosen clip, at this stage students are asked to make these exchanges comprehensible to the TT audience, while remaining respectful of all involved figures. It is now that the teacher must dedicate some time to a brief but complete tutorial on translational strategies (Pedersen, 2005; Ramière, 2006: 156–7). The extreme delicacy of this operation lies in the necessity to translate from one culture to another, respecting the restrictions imposed by these means, which, according to Hatim and Mason (1997: 65–6), include "the shift in mode from speech to writing", "physical constraints of available space [...] and the pace of the sound track dialogue", "the reduction of the source text", and "the requirement of matching the visual image". The nature of these restrictions will most likely lead students to reduce their use of extensive explanations, which in standard translational exercises, on the contrary, are treated (and at times abused) as the most immediate translational strategy, above all in difficult or embarrassing cases (Olk, 2002). The amount of factors to be considered, both from a linguistic-cultural standpoint and from a technical perspective creates another opportunity for intercultural skills acquisition, given that it postulates both a critical evaluation of the available possibilities and subsequently, once a choice is made, a definitive assumption of personal responsibility. These skills, both required and further developed by the activity, concern the final component which, according to Byram (1997: 63–4), constitutes intercultural competence, "critical cultural awareness".

5.5. Editing

From an educational perspective, this final stage is dedicated to reflection on the process which has been undertaken and on what has been learned. However, continuing with the simulation of AVT work, this stage can here be labelled "editing", since all operations carried out by the professional subtitler at this point are easily translatable into educational activities aimed at intercultural competence. In this final phase, undertaken slowly and meticulously, individually or in small groups, students evaluate their own work and that of their peers by breaking the subtitled text down into minimal temporal sequences from the following perspectives related to the subtitled video:

- Author and text: Do the subtitles respect the film as regards length, time on the screen, etc.? As far as lexical choice, syntax, etc.? Is it possible to assimilate the model reader of the TT to that of the ST? What would the director think of the subtitles produced?
- Source text culture: Is the image given by the written text to the target audience realistic? Does it respect differences and peculiarities?
- Target text culture: Are subtitles easy to read? Can the TT audience easily relate to the film through them without forgetting the film's original cultural context? Will the TT audience consequently react to the text in a similar manner to the ST audience?

On a methodological level, so that each student can make the most constructive use of their multiple responsibilities during revision, it is opportune to carry out this activity individually at first (or within the group that has written the subtitles). As before (section 5.2.), it is possible to use analytical worksheets either prepared in large part by the teacher or assigned to the students to design on the basis of the three above-mentioned factors. After they have seen and analysed their clip several times, making necessary changes to the subtitled text, the groups can exchange clips and repeat this analysis using the work of their peers. Alternatively, three student "panels" can be formed; each specialized in one of the three principal subtitling relationships, who judge all the subtitled clips produced by the activity. Whatever the method used at this stage, it is important to leave ample time for collective comments and discussion. Ideally, at the end of the process, projection of the clip to other classes who were not involved in the project can be organized, so that the students/subtitlers can receive feedback from the TT audience itself that they envisioned during their work.

6. Conclusions

This study can only conclude in the hope that this exploratory review will soon be succeeded by experimental research which concretely verifies the efficiency of subtitle creation in the acquisition of intercultural competence in the foreign language classroom. This possibility becomes even more intriguing given the existence of certain strong analogies between the subtitling process intended as a combination of reflection and technical-translational operations and the principles of Intercultural Foreign Language Education: the typical roles and responsibilities of the intercultural mediator assumed by individual subtitling; the need for students, as a direct result of this role, to investigate the ST culture with curiosity and humility, whilst reflecting on their own base cultures; the importance of dedicating attention to the totality of non-verbal codes that accompany speech in defining the meaning of the overall message; the cultural relativity of the message; the direct experience of language as a cultural product and, at the same time, as a complex phenomenon to be linked to the confines of technical and/or cultural constraints etc. These similarities have been uncovered largely as a result of the analytical tools offered by Cultural Studies. The order of reflections such affinities have generated seems to foreshadow a fruitful future application of methodologies tied to the creation of subtitles alongside those activities already considered apt for the integral promotion of linguistic and intercultural competence in the foreign language classroom.

References

Bartrina, F., and E. Espasa (2005), Audiovisual Translation. In M. Tennent (ed.), *Training for the New Millennium*. Amsterdam: John Benjamins, 83–100.
Barker, C. (2004), *The SAGE Dictionary of Cultural Studies*. London: SAGE.
Bassnett, S. (2003), The Translation Turn in Cultural Studies. In S. Petrilli (ed.), *Translation, Translation*. Amsterdam: Rodopi, 433–49.

Borghetti, C. (2008), Un modello metodologico per l'insegnamento interculturale della lingua straniera. Dalla pratica didattica alla generazione teorica. PhD thesis. National University of Ireland, Galway.

Brisset. A. (2003), Alterity in Translation: An Overview of Theories and Practices. In S. Petrilli (ed.), *Translation, Translation*. Amsterdam: Rodopi, 101–32.

Brown, A. L., and J. C. Campione (1994), Guided Discovery in a Community of Learners. In K. McGilly (ed.), *Classroom Lessons: Integrating Cognitive Theory and Classroom Practice*. Cambridge (MA): The MIT Press, 229–70.

Byram, M. (1988), Foreign Language Education and Cultural Studies. *Language, Culture and Curriculum* 1(1), 15–31.

—(1989), *Cultural Studies in Foreign Language Education*. Clevedon: Multilingual Matters.

—(1997), *Teaching and Assessing Intercultural Communicative Competence*. Clevedon: Multilingual Matters.

—(2000), Assessing Intercultural Competence in Language Teaching. *Sprogforum* 18(6). <http://inet.dpb.dpu.dk/infodok/sprogforum/Espr18/byram.html> (accessed 04/02/2011).

— (2008), *From Foreign Language Education to Education for Intercultural Citizenship. Essays and Reflections*. Clevedon: Multilingual Matters.

Byram, M., and G. Zarate (1994), *Definitions, Objectives and Assessment of Socio-Cultural Competence*. Strasbourg: Council of Europe.

Caimi, A. (2006), Audiovisual Translation and Language Learning: The Promotion of Interlingual Subtitles. *The Journal of Specialised Translation* 6, 85–98.

Calvani, A. (1998), Costruttivismo, progettazione didattica e tecnologie. In D. Bramanti (ed.), *Progettazione formativa e valutazione*. Roma: Carocci, 43–58.

Clifford, J. (1986), Introduction: Partial Truths. In J. Clifford and G. E. Marcus (eds), *Writing Culture: the Poetics and Politics of Ethnography*. Berkeley: University of California Press.

Deardorff, D. K. (2006), Identification and Assessment of Intercultural Competence as a Student Outcome of Internalization. *Journal of Studies in International Education* 10(3), 241–66.

During, S. (2005), *Cultural Studies: A Critical Introduction*. New York: Routledge.

Eco, U. (2004), *Lector in fabula: la cooperazione interpretativa nei testi narrativi*. Nona edizione. Milano: Tascabili Bompiani.

Gambier, Y. (2006), Multimodality in Audiovisual Translation. In M. Carroll, H. Gerzymisch-Arbogast and S. Nauert (eds), *Audiovisual Translation Scenarios: Proceedings of the Marie Curie Euroconferences MuTra: Audiovisual Translation Scenarios*. Copenhagen, 1–5 May, 91–8.

Geertz, C. (1973), *The Interpretation of Culture*. New York: Basic Books.

Gottlieb, H. (2004), Language-Political Implications of Subtitling. In P. Orero (ed.), *Topics in Audiovisual Translation*. Amsterdam: John Benjamins, 83–100.

Guilherme, M. (2002), *Critical Citizens for an Intercultural World: Foreign Language Education as Cultural Politics*. Clevedon: Multilingual Matters.

Hadzilacos, T., S. Papadakis and S. Sokoli (2004), Learner's Version of Professional Environment: Film Subtitling as an ICTE Tool for Foreign Language Learning. In J. Nall and R. Robson (eds), *Proceedings of World Conference on E-Learning in Corporate, Government, Healthcare, and Higher Education 2004*. Chesapeake, VA: AACE, 680–5.

Hatim, B., and I. Mason (1997), *The Translator as Communicator*. London: Routledge.

Izzo, C. (1970), Responsabilità del traduttore, ovvero esercizio di umiltà. In C. Izzo (ed.), *Civiltà Britannica, vol. II, Impressioni e note*. Roma: Edizioni di storia e letteratura, 377–99.

Jonassen, D. H. (1994), Thinking Technology. Toward a Constructivist Design Model. *Educational Technology* 34(4), 34–7.

Katan, D. (1999), *Translating Cultures*. Manchester: St. Jerome.

——(2009), Translator Training and Intercultural Competence. In S. Cavagnoli, E. Di Giovanni and R. Merlini (eds), *La ricerca nella comunicazione interlinguistica. Modelli teorici e metodologici*. Milano: FrancoAngeli, 282–301.

Kramsch, C. (1993), *Context and Culture in Language Teaching*. Oxford: Oxford University Press.

——(1998), The Privilege of the Intercultural Speaker. In M. Byram and M. Fleming (eds), *Language Teaching in Intercultural Perspective. Approaches Through Drama and Ethnography*. Cambridge: Cambridge University Press, 16–31.

Krashen, S. (1985), *The Input Hypothesis: Issues and Implications*. London: Longman.

Lázár, I. (2007), *Developing and Assessing Intercultural Communicative Competence. A Guide for Language Teachers and Teachers Educators*. Strasbourg: Council of Europe.

Lutter, C., and M. Reisenleitner (2002), *Cultural Studies. Eine Einführung*, Vienna: Erhard Löcker Gesmbh.

McLoughlin, L., and J. Lertola (forthcoming), Sottotitolando s'impara: la sottotitolazione come ausilio all'apprendimento linguistico. *Italiano L2 in classe*. Florence: Mondadori.

Morini, M. (2007), *La traduzione: teorie, strumenti, pratiche*. Milano: Sironi.

Neves, J. (2004), Language Awareness through Training in Subtitling. In P. Orero (ed.), *Topics in Audiovisual Translation*. Amsterdam: John Benjamins, 127–40.

Niemeier, S. (1991), Intercultural Dimensions of Pragmatics in Film Synchronisation. In J. Blommaert and J. Verschueren (eds), *The Pragmatics of International and Intercultural Communication*. Amsterdam: John Benjamins, 145–62.

Olk, H. M. (2002), Transalting Culture – A Think-aloud Protocol Study. *Language Teaching Research* 6(2), 121–44.

Palincsar, A. S., and A. L. Brown (1984), Reciprocal Teaching of Comprehension-Fostering and Comprehension Monitoring Activities. *Cognition and Instruction* 1(2), 117–75.

Pavesi, M. (2002), Sottotitoli: dalla semplificazione nella traduzione all'apprendimento linguistico. In A. Caimi (ed.), *RILA – Rassegna Italiana di Linguistica Applicata* 34(1–2). Special issue *Cinema: Paradiso delle Lingue. I sottotitoli nell'apprendimento linguistico*, 127–42.

Pedersen, J. (2005), How is Culture Rendered in Subtitles? In: *MuTra – Challenges of Multidimensional Translation: Conference Proceedings*. <http://www.euroconferences.info/proceedings/2005_Proceedings/2005_Pedersen_Jan.pdf> (accessed 04/02/2011).

Pinto, D. (2010), Lost in Subtitle Translations: The Case of Advice in the English Subtitles of Spanish Films. *Intercultural Pragmatics* 7(2), 257–77.

Pym, A. (2010), *Translation and Text Transfer. An Essay on the Principles of Intercultural Communication*. Tarragona: Intercultural Studies Group.

Ramière, N. (2006), Reaching a Foreign Audience: Cultural Transfers in Audiovisual Translation. *The Journal of Specialised Translation* 6, 152–66.

Rogers, M. (2008), Translation and Foreign Language Learning. A Synergistic Exploration of Research Problems. In H. P. Krings and F. Mayer (eds), *Sprachenvielfalt im Kontext von Fachkommunikation, Übersetzung und Fremdsprachenunterricht*. Berlin: Frank & Timme, 117–27.

Sokoli, S. (2006), Learning via Subtitling (LvS): A Tool for the Creation of Foreign Language Learning Activities Based on Film Subtitling. In M. Carroll, H. Gerzymisch-Arbogast and S. Nauert (eds), *Audiovisual Translation Scenarios: Proceedings of the Marie Curie Euroconferences MuTra: Audiovisual Translation Scenarios*. Copenhagen, 1–5 May, 66–73.

Talaván Zanón, N. (2006), Using Subtitles to Enhance Foreign Language Learning. *Porta Linguarum* 6, 41–52.

Venuti, L. (1995), *The Translator's Invisibility: A History of Translation*. London: Routledge.

Williams, H., and D. Thorne (2000), The Value of Teletext Subtiling as a Medium for Language Learning. *System* 28, 217–28.

MARCELLA DE MARCO

Bringing Gender into the Subtitling Classroom

1. Introduction

The increase in publications on Audiovisual Translation (AVT) experienced in recent years reflects an increase in the range of research paths that this field has been able to generate, as well as of the innumerable applications and interconnections that it may establish with other disciplines. Through the studies of Neves (2005, 2008), Bernal-Merino (2006, 2007), Orero (2007), Vercauteren (2007), Remael et al. (2008) we have widened our knowledge beyond the mere linguistic and technical aspects which concern dubbing, subtitling, voice-over and the other audiovisual translation modes. It has therefore been possible to see how the study and use of these modes may be adapted to the needs of increasingly heterogeneous audiences and to the challenges posed by an ever-changing technology. At the same time, a parallel interest in the didactics of AVT has grown as a consequence of both the more established status that translation degrees enjoy in higher education (HE), and the need to help students to acquire a highly special-ized profile in order to meet the new expectations of the current profes-sional market. Consequently, many pedagogical considerations on how to achieve this objective have been raised (Tennent, 2005; Díaz-Cintas, 2008; Arumí Ribas and Romero Fresco, 2008).

The interdisciplinary nature of AVT has also surfaced thanks to scholars who have pointed out its cultural and sociological impact on the audiences' perception of audiovisual programmes and, at the same time, the extent to which AVT may be conditioned by cultural and social con-straints (Delabastita, 1989; Díaz-Cintas, 1997; Santamaria, 2001). One of the recent research areas to highlight this multifaceted nature is that which explores gender within and through AVT (De Marco, 2006, 2008, 2009). Through an in-depth analysis of a number of North American and British films and of its dubbed and subtitled translations into Spanish and Italian, it has been observed that the ways in which films are dubbed and/ or subtitled may contribute to encouraging (or preventing) the reinforcement of gender stereotypes and prejudices in the way people think and behave. The more sexist and homophobic nuances identified in some of the dubbed/subtitled versions of the exchanges analysed have shown that AVT plays a prominent role in the creation of stereotyping and denigration, thus running the risk of favouring the interests of certain sectors of society to the detriment of others.

These studies – some of the first to have explored gender issues in AVT – were aimed at awakening people's awareness of the constant presence of gender in the audiovisual programmes which crowd our eyes and minds on a daily basis and of the fact that we are passive recipients of and, to a certain extent, are also responsible for the way in which certain sexual, social and ethnic groups are represented on the screen. Consequently we may also become responsible for the way in which they are perceived and treated in our society. The way in which we see and interpret films – as spectators – mediate their linguistic transfer – as AV professionals – and investigate this transfer – as scholars – is, in most cases, the result of an interculturally shared background composed of values, habits and bias that we have unconsciously assimilated. However, despite the difficulty of accepting that things may be interpreted or done differently, as active players in the society in which we live, we have a duty to question unfair social dynamics which perpetuate social injustice. It is such a dynamic that keeps gender binaries alive.

This paper has been written as a result of this social and academic commitment. As a scholar in Gender Studies and Audiovisual Translation, and as a lecturer in Translation, I feel responsible for actively participating in the eradication of gender-biased language through the work I perform every day. I have therefore explored the ways in which gender and identity-related issues may be integrated within the curriculum of the subtitling module that I coordinate and teach for the Master's Degree in Applied Translation Studies (MA ATS) at London Metropolitan University (LMU).

2. Gender and education

Gender (and its interrelations with ethnicity, sexuality and class) has been thoroughly explored in the last thirty years from many different angles and in different contexts: Film Studies (Mulvey, 1975), Post-colonial Studies (Spivak, 1990), Translation Studies (Godayol, 2000), Sociolinguistics (Coates, 2004) and Education (Pitman, 2008). This variety of gender perspectives has become the subject of many courses offered in degrees in Social Sciences with the number of courses on offer having significantly increased in the last few years. This shows a need to transmit – on the part of some teachers – and to receive/widen – on the part of some students – their knowledge on such a relevant aspect of everyone's identity, in determining the roles that men and women play or are asked to play because of their gender. However, such an encouraging interest from many social spheres does not seem to be accompanied by a real commitment, on the part of the institutions, to embark on concrete initiatives which will ultimately result in the actual overthrow of gender bias and, therefore, in the achievement of a more balanced society. Many academics have denounced the persistence of racialized, male-centred criteria still in play in all spheres of education which regulate, for example, the admission and assessment of students, and govern the kind of teaching material to be delivered (Clarricoates, 1987; Delamont, 1990; Barres, 2006). Focusing our attention on what happens in the HE environment; Quinn (2003, in Burke, 2006: 89) argues that "although women's participation in higher education has dramatically increased, the curriculum has largely stayed the same". On the subject of the lifelong learning policy as it is currently formulated in the UK, Leathwood (2006: 52) adds that:

> [W]here gendered patterns are recognized, these are constructed as a matter of individual choice, hence again shifting the responsibility onto the individual [...]. Social inclusion is framed in terms of an unquestioning inclusion within a highly stratified and unequal labour market, with little in the policy texts suggesting a commitment to lifelong learning for an active, creative and critical citizenship.

As a consequence, although the British HE policy seems to be keen to emphasize the importance of promoting employability through proper training and support,

> the discourse of employability ignores gender, ethnicity, social class and other markers of identity that impact on students' experience and entry to the labour market. Where lifelong learning activities are directed at producing "employable" subjects, they are also reproducing the gendered (as well as classed and racialized) worker identities of the labour market. [...] The lifelong learner is therefore constructed as a compliant employable subject, able to fit into the existing gendered, classed and racialized social order, rather than a critical thinker and citizen. (Morley, 2001 in Leathwood, 2006: 48–9)

The HE policy applied in the last ten years in the universities in the UK has placed much emphasis on the need to equip students with key skills, i.e. communication, numeracy, the use of information technology and learning how to learn (Recommendation 19 of the Dearing Report);[1] skills which are seen as essential "to contribute to wealth generation" (Adams, 2007: 97). Other concepts which this policy seems to insist on are: widening students' participation through fair access and raising aspirations, development of learning as a two-way process between tutors and students and development of critical thinking through the promotion of challenging tasks which resemble real-life tasks. All these recommendations appear very challenging and are actually forcing HE staff to revise their roles as educators and ·the ways they are supposed to deliver knowledge. However, many scholars have identified contradictions and gaps between the theoretical relevance of these principles and their practical application, and question the fact that this is seen as a straightforward, neutral process which does little to

---

1   The Dearing Report published in 1997 includes a set of 93 recommendations regarding the funding and expansion of HE standards. Although it has often received a number of complaints and critiques mainly due to the introduction of the obligation for undergraduates to contribute to the costs of their studies, it has to be acknowledged that the new policy which has come into force has brought education closer to the professional environment. For a more extensive overview of these recommendations see Watson and Amoah (2007).

promote alternative thinking about the social construction of students' and tutors' experiences. They point out that knowledge is not neutral and that creating knowledge means creating "skills and understanding that makes sense of the world and help people to act upon it collectively in order to change it for the better" (Tett, 2006: 105). It has also been stressed that participation does not translate only into issues of access and of raising aspirations and that students' aspirations cannot be decontextualized from their social positioning (Burke, 2006: 89).

This overview of the debates surrounding the discourse on gender in relation to the HE landscape shows that it is in the classroom that problems of social discrimination and marginalization easily come into play. Consequently, this represents the best arena for raising awareness of these problems and perhaps for them to be addressed by trained professionals. What is less clear is how to concretely succeed in raising this awareness, how to convey to students the understanding of why such awareness is so important and how to make it usable for them in their life beyond university. Through this paper I have tried to address these questions, attempted to give an answer and suggested some recommendations for further improvement.

3. Gender in the subtitling classroom

Whatever the route students decide to embark upon when entering university, one activity they are expected to participate in is academic writing. Burke (2006) points out that academic writing courses should be organized in such a way that students are made aware of the contribution that they could bring to meaning-making through their writing. In this way she trusts that they "could also contribute to challenging hegemonic academic practices within universities that serve to maintain privilege and exclusion" (ibid: 91). If students studying for scientific degrees are able to contribute to meaning-making, then this is all the more feasible for students attending translation courses. Translation is, first and foremost, the transfer of a message contained in a text, but it is also an interpretation and, therefore, a personal (re)construction of that meaning. When we teach students to identify translation problems and to devise specific strategies accordingly, what we are doing is helping them to understand *how* the information is constructed in the source text in order to decide *how* it has to be rendered in order to be intelligible for the target readership (or audience in the case of audiovisual texts). The social and political constraints that govern this *how* are often unknown or pass unnoticed, hence the blind acceptance of those constraints and the perpetuation of the bias inherent in them. The awareness of how many subtle nuances hiding well-rooted stereotypes appear in cinematographic language and in its translations is what I have tried to awaken in the students attending the above-mentioned subtitling module. Before describing how I put this into practice I will briefly outline the MA framework in which this module is integrated.

3.1. Framework

By offering a wide range of language pathways (twenty-four), the MA ATS at London Metropolitan University has always encouraged the participation of "non-traditional" students, i.e. students who are "far more mixed in terms of age and educational, class, cultural and linguistic background" (Warren, 2002: 86–7). The subtitling module[2] is aimed at further widening the choice of disciplines offered to these students, thus allowing them to specialize in a field which is increasingly expanding and to acquire a kind of knowledge that they could make use of in their native countries or in the UK. This is a designate, in-class module offered in the second semester after the completion of four other core modules which are meant to

2   The need to introduce subtitling on the Master's was dictated by the fact that an increased number of our students had their work placements in subtitling companies in the years preceding the design of this module in 2007. It ran for the first time in the academic year 2008–9.

provide students with a solid and varied background: theoretical notions, an overview of the range of non-literary translations in existence (legal, medical, advertising), and computer literacy (use of translation memories). These modules are therefore seen as preparation for acquiring the right familiarity with both theoretical and technological issues which students will be faced with in the subtitling module.

3.2. Gender training in subtitling training

Bearing in mind the dictates of HE policy mentioned in the previous section, the main objectives which have been established in building up the structure of this module have been: choice of appropriate software that meets the requirements of the subtitling industry and selection of relevant topics and activities resembling real-life tasks. In order to promote both practical and critical skills, the teaching sessions are structured in one hour-long lecture and one hour-long seminar, the former introducing the theoretical topic of the week which will constitute the basis of the homework to be assigned, and the latter being based upon discussion – in pairs and with the tutor – of the homework assigned the week before, which is always carried out with the use of the software.

When deciding the topics of the teaching sessions and the homework to be assigned the central question was: "*What is most important for these students to know and what might be the best ways for them to learn it?*" (Toohey, 1999: 25, emphasis in the original). Of course, as this was the first time that this module ran, my focus was on ensuring that they would gain a practical command of the essential techniques of subtitling practice so that, when they enter the subtitling industry, they will have possibly developed an awareness of the linguistic, cultural, semiotic and technological factors inherent in this kind of translation. From this perspective, special emphasis has been placed on a sequence of increasingly difficult activities: from warm-up tasks aimed at familiarizing students with the software, to more complicated ones aimed at producing short intralingual transcriptions through to more advanced ones aimed at creating longer interlingual translations in the form of subtitles which are appropriately synchronized with images and soundtrack.

How does gender fit into this organization which does not seem to differ greatly from the one implemented in other universities? When I began to think of the possibility of including gender in my curriculum, my first idea was to introduce it as one of the many other topics dealt with throughout the twelve-week course that I would be presenting in the form of a lecture followed by the usual discussion. However, as such it would have appeared to be just another content option that would remain quite disconnected from the rest of the more technical subjects presented each week (spatial and temporal constraints, stylistic conventions, culture-boundness in subtitling etc.) and which would probably have been seen by most students as marginal and not really having a bearing on subtitling practice. I therefore decided to keep the gender lecture for the last session of the course, but in the meantime – from week four onwards – I assigned them tasks involving the translation of clips containing hints for gender discussion (sexist remarks, common swear words, not particularly offensive exchanges in the source text which have been translated into homophobic innuendoes in some target languages). I did not provide a reason for that choice, and this allowed me to gauge the students' awareness of the gender-biased expressions characterizing everyday language and their capacity to identify them and to make a conscious decision on whether and how to reproduce them in their own language. Most of the students' translations were literal subtitles which had been properly spotted and synchronized. No significant remarks were made by them during our weekly discussions on the homework assigned, and this prompted me to design a questionnaire (Table 19) which I finally presented in the last week before delivering my presentation on gender in AVT.

Table 19: Questionnaire provided in the last session

---

1) What, in your opinion, was the point of the assignment?

2) What does gender represent for you?

3) How is gender identity perceived in your own country?

4) Did you think that gender would be an issue when dealing with AVT problems?

5) Do you think that the way you perceive gender (your own and others') may affect your professional activity as a translator? If so, in what sense?

6) Do you think that developing a sensitivity to gender issues during the educational years will help you develop your professional identity, and if so why?

7) To what extent do you think that awareness of gender issues may be relevant to AVT professionals?

8) Do you perceive AVT as a means which enhances or limits the perpetuation of gender bias?

Only a minority (one out of eight students attending the session) understood the real intent of that homework.[3] Most of them saw it as a challenging activity aimed at developing their capacity to deal with slang and colloquial register in subtitling. A few just considered it another exercise to further practice condensation and other subtitling techniques but they did not perceive the socio-cultural subtext intrinsic to the clips. It

---

3   The low number of students is due to the fact that, as already mentioned, this is an elective module. Moreover, their selection is also dependent on the availability of native-speaking tutors who work outside the university. I am aware that because of this slender range of respondents, the interpretation of the findings might appear somewhat anecdotal. It is worth pointing out that this has been one of the first experiments aimed at introducing a socio-ideological topic in the teaching of a very technological discipline. The strengths and weaknesses in the way this exercise has been carried out will be certainly taken into consideration for a more thorough implementation of this approach in the near future.

is interesting to see that the majority skated around the second question: instead of clearly explaining what gender was for them, they answered that they found it more or less important.[4] Some considered it relevant only in grammar, others "important in life but not while working". More sensible answers were given to question three regarding the situation in their own countries, although some of their opinions appeared, to some extent, contradictory.[5] The most relevant findings are reflected in the answers to the last questions. Only three of them suspected, before they started the subtitling course, that gender would be an issue and that developing sensitivity about it in the academic environment would help them in their future professional life. The others did not think about this (or this idea "had only just crossed their minds") and considered gender a private thing that has nothing to do with work. Two of them considered that awareness of these issues may be relevant to AVT professionals, another two did not agree and the rest thought that it depends on the professional's own gender. As regards the last point, only two students thought that AVT may have a role in enhancing or limiting the perpetuation of gender bias, but that the producers' intentions and the societal attitudes must also be considered. The remaining students were unsure or did not answer.

What this picture shows is that, although on the one hand there is sensitivity and interest in discovering to what extent AVT may affect, or may be affected by, the presence of identity-related factors, on the other hand the link between everyday life and work does not seem so obvious. Is work not part and parcel of everyday life? If – sticking with one of the previous answers – gender is present in grammar and lexicon, is it not also present in the grammar and lexicon of the language we use in our daily (private and professional) exchanges? Part of this gap was filled after I showed

---

4   The vagueness of the students' answers might be a direct consequence of the breadth of question two, which could be interpreted in many different ways. This question will be revised and made more specific.

5   Some Polish students argued that men and women are treated equally in Poland, but they also stated that "women are considered more fragile, which, in some cases, may be discriminatory".

students the professional translations into Italian and Spanish of some of the clips they themselves had subtitled. Their surprise at seeing the more sexist or more neutral renderings on display made them see more clearly what the point of the questionnaire, the lecture and the brainstorming we had just had was.

3.3. Suggestions for further improvements

These reactions have enabled me to identify the pros and cons of the method used to bring gender awareness into the subtitling classroom and, therefore, to suggest some improvements which could be implemented for the future. The fact that I have introduced this topic in a very technology-based module has certainly made it easier for me to understand the students' approach in dealing with aspects of translation/subtitling which do not directly interest the technical and linguistic sphere. Their curiosity to see, in the last session, how different the perception of a dialogue exchange may be when words are charged with additional (offensive) innuendoes proves that gender has been perceived not simply as one of the topics that makes up the course syllabus, but as something which may conspicuously impact on the audience, and therefore to be taken into account. I am not entirely convinced, however, that the students have been put in a position to really understand how much they can use this awareness in their life as (AVT) professionals. In order for them to see how much they can bring by way of their translations, they must first understand how gender manifests itself in social life. This will take time, and it means that they should be faced more often with tasks containing gender challenges, thus enabling them to assimilate the topic and see it as an integral part of their identity which also manifests itself in their work. From this point of view, a more gradual distribution of this subject in different sessions would allow me to test the students' reactions before "knowing" about gender, how their awareness changes throughout the course after they are faced with this reality and whether this change results in a change in the way they approach their translation tasks.

This idea of rationing the transfer of knowledge is what Bruner (1977) calls "spiral curriculum", that is a curriculum in which topics should "be developed and redeveloped in later grades" (ibid.: 54). His assumptions about the usefulness of structuring the subjects to be taught in such a way apply to the discourse of primary education where emphasis is placed on the fact that children need to be exposed at an early age to the ideas and styles that in their later life will make them into educated people. However, it is readily possible to extrapolate this approach to the case of the teaching of gender – and of any other socio-cultural phenomenon – in a mainly technological context such as the subtitling university classroom. This could be identified as "nonspecific transfer of training", i.e. "the transfer of principles and attitudes" as opposed to the "specific" one referring to the transferable skills, to "its specific applicability to tasks that are highly similar to those we originally learned to perform" (ibid. 17).

What I have attempted to do through the experiment described in this paper is to combine the specific transfer – of technical and linguistic skills essential to subtitling practice – with the non-specific transfer of "great issues, principles, and values that a society deems worthy of the continual concern of its members" (ibid.: 52). I see these principles as strictly integral to translation, in general, and to subtitling in particular. This way of instilling knowledge and sensitivity is the most fruitful method of ensuring that students continue to learn, i.e. not only the capacity to use the skills acquired in education in order to recognize and solve technical problems which resemble the ones they have mastered during their training, but also the capacity to understand what the implications of carrying out their tasks might be when the representation of (their) gender is at stake. Structurewise, this method proves to be very successful. The only hurdle lies in the duration of the course analysed. As previously stressed, the subtitling module taught at LMU lasts for twelve weeks. Introducing gender through the "spiral curriculum" approach would mean that most of the sessions would end up revolving around gender, and it would thus take control over the entire module. Like many similar subtitling courses run in other universities, this one relies on the weekly use of software. Consequently, half course is based upon building up the students' confidence with this tool as well as on enhancing their familiarity with technical and stylistic conventions and working issues. The "spiral curriculum" would certainly be more effective if, rather than a twelve-week module, it were a one-year course. Developing the gender topic across different AVT modes would prove more fruitful still. On a larger temporal scale, the many facets of gender analysis (gender as a concept, as social roles, as projection of stereotypes, as an ethical issue affecting the translator's performance etc.) could be integrated in this course more successfully. Gender issues would be introduced, for example, every two or three weeks. By the end of the course the students would have acquired full awareness of how much gender issues might affect the ethics of their profession.

4. Conclusions

Use of information technology, the student-tutor relationship as a two-way process, the development of awareness and critical thinking, and the provision of real-life tasks are the key principles promoted by the HE policy. They are all reflected in the teaching of the subtitling module offered at LMU as well as, very probably, in many other UK and international institutions. What I have shown in this paper is how these principles can be adapted to aspects of the teaching/learning of subtitling practice which go beyond the technical and linguistic domains. Teaching subtitling, nowadays, means, first of all, transmitting the skills necessary to cope with spatial and temporal constraints. For this purpose, much emphasis is placed on the development of students' expertise in the use of technology, on which professional subtitlers have become increasingly dependent in recent years.

However, the idea governing the setting up of the topics presented in the subtitling module, which has been taken as a reference in this paper, is that "training subtitlers is a socialization process [and] learning to translate is basically learning how to cope with constraints, social and other"

152 MARCELLA DE MARCO

(Kovačič, 1995, in Kruger, 2008: 80). I would like to stress the value of these "social" and "other" constraints contained in the aforementioned quotation. By "constraints" both Kovačič and Kruger mainly refer to the linguistic (lack of knowledge of a foreign language) and sensorial (lack of or reduced sight/hearing) hurdles which some spectators experience and which force AV professionals to acquire specific training in order to find the right balance between the norms of written and spoken language. However, from the sociologists' perspective, socialization is essentially the process by which people acquire the habits and skills necessary to participate and act in their society. What I have tried to bring to my students within the subtitling classroom is a "social" and "Other" understanding, i.e. awareness that the work they produce in class and, later on, into their work environment makes part of this process of socialization. When they translate they can either bring in their translations the values, the symbols and the shared stereotypes of the culture to which they belong, or try to question those values and symbols if they think they fail to represent themselves. Subtitling is a matter of technical constraints but, just as in all kinds of translation, also involves a construction of meaning and decisions. Making meaning also means making sensible decisions about the possibility of challenging hegemonic practices which can still be found in all workplaces.[6] By describing the way in which Bruner's (1997) "spiral curriculum" approach has been implemented in part, and could be implemented further, to raise awareness of gender-related topics, this paper attempts to suggest to other scholars involved in the training of the newer generations of subtitlers a pedagogical approach which will hopefully result in the training not of "compliant" but of critical employable subjects.

6   It is important to stress at this point that when it comes to instilling awareness of identity-related issues, the delivery of the teaching in class tends to be more fruitful than in the case of distance learning since the physical presence of the tutor within a close space forces the students to express their own views and concerns about these issues.

References

Adams, J., and D. Watson (2007), Higher Education, Knowledge Economy: From Robbins to "the Gathering Storm". In D. Watson and M. Amoah (eds), *The Dearing Report: Ten Years On*. London: Institute of Education, University of London, 81–108.

Arumí Ribas, M., and P. Romero Fresco (2008), A Practical Proposal for the Training of Respeakers 1. *The Journal of Specialised Translation* 10, 106–27.

Barres, B. (2006), Does Gender Matter? *Nature* 442, 133–6.

Bernal-Merino, M. (2006), On the Translation of Video Games. *The Journal of Specialised Translation*, 6, 22–36.

——(2007), What's in a Game? *Localisation Focus* 6(1), 19–31.

Bruner, J. (1977), *The Process of Education*. Cambridge, MA: Harward University Press.

Burke, P. (2006), Fair Access? Exploring Gender, Access and Participation Beyond Entry to Higher Education. In C. Leathwood and B. Francis (eds), *Gender and Lifelong Learning. Critical Feminist Engagements*. London: Routledge, 83–93.

Clarricoates, K. (1987), Dinosaurs in the Classroom: The "Hidden" Curriculum in Primary Schools. In M. Arnot and G. Weiner (eds), *Gender and the Politics of Schooling*. London: Hitchinson, 155–65.

Coates, J. (2004), *Women, Men and Language: A Sociolinguistic Account of Gender Differences in Language*, 3rd edn. Harlow: Pearson Longman.

Delabastita, D. (1989), Translation and Mass-Communication: Film and TV Translation as Evidence of Cultural Dynamics. *Babel* 35(4), 193–218.

Delamont, S. (1990), *Sex Roles and the School*. London: Methuen.

De Marco, M. (2006), Audiovisual Translation from a Gender Perspective. *The Journal of Specialised Translation* 6, 167–84.

——(2008), *Gender Stereotypes and Dubbing: Similarities and Differences in the Translation of Hollywood and British Films*. Vic: Universidad de Vic. PhD Dissertation.

——(2009), Gender Portrayal in Dubbed and Subtitled Comedies. In J. Díaz-Cintas (ed.), *New Trends in Audiovisual Translation* Bristol: Multilingual Matters, 176–94.

Díaz-Cintas, J. (1997), *El subtitulado en tanto que modalidad de traducción fílmica dentro del marco teórico de los estudios sobre traducción* (Misterioso asesinato en Manhattan, *Woody Allen, 1993*). Valencia: Universidad de Valencia. PhD Dissertation.

—— (ed.) (2008), *The Didactics of Audiovisual Translation*. Amsterdam: John Benjamins.

Godayol, P. (2000), *Spazi di frontiera. Genere e traduzione*. Translated by Annarita Taronna. Bari: Palomar, 2002.

Kovačič, I. (1995), Reinforcing or Changing Norms in Subtitling. In C. Dollerup and V. Appel (eds), *Teaching Translation and Interpreting 3: New Horizons*. Amsterdam: John Benjamins, 105–9.

Kruger, J. (2008), Subtitler Training as Part of a General Training Programme in the Language Professions. In J. Díaz-Cintas (ed.), *The Didactics of Audiovisual Translation*. Amsterdam: John Benjamins, 71–87.

Leathwood, C. (2006), Gendered Constructions of Lifelong Learning and the Learner in the UK Policy Context. In C. Leathood and B. Francis (eds), *Gender and Lifelong Learning. Critical Feminist Engagements*. London: Routledge, 40–53.

—— (2007), Gender Equity in Post-Secondary Education. In C. Skelton, B. Francis and L. Smulyan (eds), *Handbook of Gender and Education*. London: Sage, 166–78.

Morley, L. (2001), Producing New Workers: Quality, Equality and Employability in Higher Education. *Quality in Higher Education* 7(2), 131–8.

Mulvey, L. (1975), Visual Pleasure and Narrative Cinema. In A. Kaplan (ed.), *Feminism and Film* (2000). New York: Oxford University Press, 34–47.

Neves, J. (2005), *Audiovisual Translation: Subtitling for the Deaf and Hard-of-Hearing*. London: University of Surrey Roehampton. PhD Dissertation.

—— (2008), 10 Fallacies about Subtitling for the d/Deaf and the Hard of Hearing. *The Journal of Specialised Translation* 10, 128–43.

Orero, P. (2007), The Audio Description of a Spanish Phenomenon. *The Journal of Specialised Translation* 7, 164–78.

Pitman, T. (2008), Teaching Chicano/a Studies in the UK: Mobilising Hispanic Studies Students' Empathetic Responses to Promote Equality and Diversity. *Liaison Magazine* 1, 31–2.

Quinn, J. (2003), *Powerful Subjects: Are Women Really Taking over the University?* Stoke-on-Trent: Trentham Books.

Remael, A., A. De Houver and R. Vandekerckhove (2008), Intralingual Open Subtitling in Flanders: Audiovisual Translation, Linguistic Variation and Audience Needs. *The Journal of Specialised Translation* 10, 76–105.

Santamaria, L. (2001), *Subtitulació y referents culturals. La traducció com a mitjà d'acquisició de representations mentals*. Barcelona: Universidad Autónoma de Barcelona. PhD Dissertation.

Spivak, G. (1990), *The Postcolonial Critic: Interviews, Strategies, Dialogue*. London: Routledge.

Tennent, M. (ed.) (2005), *Training for the New Millennium: Pedagogies for Translation and Interpreting*. Amsterdam: John Benjamins.

Tett, L. (2006), Community Education: Participation, Risk and Desire. In C. Leathwood and B. Francis (eds), *Gender and Lifelong Learning. Critical Feminist Engagements*. London: Routledge, 97–107.

Toohey, S. (1999), *Design Courses for Higher Education*. Buckingham: Society for Research into Higher Education and Open University Press.

Vercauteren, G. (2007), Towards a European Guideline for Audio Description. In J. Díaz-Cintas, A. Remael and P. Orero (eds), *Media for All. Subtitling for the Deaf, Audio Description, and Sign Language*. Amsterdam: Rodopi, 139–50.

Warren, D. (2002), Curriculum Design in a Context of Widening Participation in Higher Education. *Arts and Humanities in Higher Education* 1(1), 85–9.

Watson, D., and M. Amoah (eds) (2007), *The Dearing Report: Ten Years On*. London: Institute of Education, University of London.

EITHNE O'CONNELL

Formal and Casual Language Learning: What Subtitles Have to Offer Minority Languages like Irish

1. Introduction

This chapter starts by offering the reader a general introduction to subtitles of various kinds. It then moves on to review international publications on research into the link between subtitled audiovisual media and language learning. The reasons underlying the usefulness of subtitled material are investigated with reference to the cognitive processing of aural/written texts and language learners of different levels, ages, nationalities, etc. The main findings of research conducted to date in this area are summarized and the potential for exploiting subtitles in both formal and informal learning environments is explored. Moving from the general to the more specific, the relevance of recent findings concerning subtitles and language learning is explored in relation to minority languages and Irish, in particular. This is discussed in terms of potential benefits to Irish language speakers and learners of various ages, backgrounds and ability were increased material subtitled in Irish to be provided by the national broadcasters.

As subtitles of various kinds have been used for different purposes and audiences at different times in different countries, it is not surprising that some confusion has arisen in relation to subtitling terminology and as a result, it seems wise to clarify the meanings of key terms used here. Perhaps the most important distinction is that between intralingual and interlingual subtitles. Interlingual subtitles refer, for example, to the translation subtitles which help us to view foreign language films in the cinema, on TV or DVD, etc. Thus standard (interlingual) subtitles for Anglophone viewers are translation subtitles in English accompanying foreign language audiovisual material. If Anglophone viewers wanting to learn Spanish watch audiovisual material with an English soundtrack, but with Spanish translation subtitles, these are referred to as reversed (interlingual) subtitles, since this combination is the opposite or reverse of what such people would normally be exposed to, namely, the Spanish soundtrack with subtitles in English.

Intralingual subtitles, on the other hand, are usually drafted to assist those who are hard-of-hearing or deaf, e.g. English teletext subtitles on a soap opera in English would be a typical example on television. Intralingual subtitles are also increasingly available on DVD and are intended primarily to improve the viewing experience of the deaf and hard-of-hearing, hence the use of the acronym, SDH (Subtitles for the Deaf and Hard of Hearing). As well as enhancing the viewing experience of the audience, these subtitles often have the secondary effect of improving the linguistic knowledge of congenitally deaf viewers. The scope here for subtitles to assist deaf people in developing linguistic knowledge and reading skills is considerable since the average deaf person leaves secondary school with the reading ability of a child of eight or nine years old. Although intended initially for the deaf or hard-of-hearing, once intralingual subtitles became widely available, it did not take long for language learners, especially intermediate and advanced learners, to realize that they could also benefit in a variety of ways if they viewed foreign language material with intralingual subtitles, i.e. were exposed to both soundtrack and subtitles in the same L2. In such cases, it can also be said that the learners are benefiting from bi-modal input. In this context, bi-modal refers to the fact that viewers engage with both aural and written versions of the language. Influenced by USA usage, intralingual SDH subtitles are increasingly referred to as captions and so, for the purposes of this chapter, captions will refer exclusively to intralingual subtitles, while the term subtitles will serve as a shorthand to mean only interlingual subtitles, whether standard or reversed. This is the approach adopted, for example, by Danan (2004).

Finally, closed captions and subtitles are encoded and must be accessed or switched on whereas their open counterparts are always visible on screen.

SDH are almost always closed and therefore do not bother those who do not require them, whereas cinema subtitles have traditionally always been open. A particularly attractive aspect of DVD technology is that an enormous range of closed soundtracks and captions and subtitles can be provided with individual viewers selecting the combinations which best suit their needs.

2. Learning opportunites with subtitles

Given a choice, many people regardless of age, would probably rather spend their time leisurely engaging with some form or other of multimedia, whether television, video, DVD, computer or game console, rather than consciously participating in some kind of tuition. Tuition, no matter how well designed and conducted, is often a little negatively associated with formal schooling and tends to suggest more work and less play, more pain than pleasure. Not so most multimedia experiences, however, which are almost always suggestive of leisure, fun and relaxation even though they may well offer lots of overt and/or covert opportunities for both formal and informal learning. Research over recent decades has shown that there is plenty of evidence that audiovisual material has much to offer in relation to native and foreign language learning, and the acquisition of a range of linguistic skills. To a certain extent, this has been understood within educational circles since the 1970s, when audiovisual language teaching methods came increasingly into vogue and even more so in the 1980s, when the emphasis placed by communicative teaching methods on authentic materials and situations resulted in teachers and learners increasingly using radio, audio tape and television, then, videotape and later still, CD, DVD etc. in the classroom environment.

Nowadays, due to the extensive range of, and easy access to, many forms of multimedia, opportunities for language learning through audiovisual media have never been so great. Although the focus here is on captions and subtitles, it must be remembered that AVT also includes dubbing. However, dubbing is not generally considered to have a significant role to play in facilitating language learning. Clearly foreign audiovisual material which has been dubbed into the viewer's first language has little to offer the learner at the purely linguistic level, although a few foreign phrases may survive the language transfer process. Nevertheless, a lot of valuable cultural information may well be encoded or interpreted in a dubbed foreign material and, at the very least, the viewer's interest in a foreign society and culture is being nurtured and developed. On that basis, dubbed material is not to be wholly discounted from a pedagogical point of view. It has a small but important contribution to play at an affective level and can ease the viewer into engagement with issues specific to the foreign culture. Moreover, in an environment where a minority language coexists closely with a much stronger one (as is the case with Irish and English in Ireland), most of the freely available audiovisual material is likely to be in the major language. In such a scenario, material dubbed into the minority language may prove to be a relatively quick and cost effective way to augment original minority language material which may be in short supply. Thus the mere fact of more material being available in the minority language, thanks to the use of dubbing, can clearly be beneficial for learners of the minority language.

But despite the huge increase in potential opportunities to develop language skills through formal and informal use of new media, many learners and teachers still show considerable scepticism and a reluctance to engage with the untapped linguistic resources that clearly exist. This scepticism and reluctance may have something to do with a deep rooted suspicion based on the perception that standard subtitles on foreign films, since they offer a translation in one language of a soundtrack in another language, effectively cancel out the beneficial effects of the foreign language audio exposure. So, despite lots of anecdotal evidence that watching subtitled foreign films can develop a whole variety of linguistic skills, many teachers still seem to think that viewing subtitled AV material in the classroom is a kind of lazy approach or even constitutes cheating (Danan, 2004: 67). For their part, some language learners, at least in countries like Ireland, where subtitles on English language television are not common, are also sceptical about potential benefits, possibly fearing becoming dependent on subtitles rather than developing their foreign language listening comprehension skills (Talaván Zanón, 2006: 42). On the other hand, the Scandinavians, for example, are anecdotally more than willing to acknowledge the propensity of English subtitles on television and in cinemas as a significant factor contributing to very good English language skills in their general populations. But even when learners are happy enough to view foreign language material in the classroom and/or at home, they still may show a reluctance to acquire specific viewing techniques which could help them to get more, linguistically, out of their leisure viewing – perhaps because they are afraid that that might just take away some of the fun during their leisure time.

In the case of foreign films and programmes with standard subtitles, there is considerable empirical evidence of linguistic benefit to be derived from viewing such material but this does not apply equally to all levels of learner. Reported benefits include improved passive, active and cross-cultural knowledge and skills. Specific improved outcomes have been reported in relation to aural comprehension, awareness of style (register, dialect, idiolect, slang), reading skills, word recognition, vocabulary acquisition, spelling, paralinguistic features, improved motivation, increased confidence, development of foreign language learning and translation strategies, including use of dictionaries etc.

For beginners, standard subtitles may function rather like dubbing, probably by helping most in terms of providing a bridge between the home and the foreign cultures. Reversed subtitles and captions, on the other hand, rarely appear appropriate for beginners. So it can be said that the main function of AVT for beginners seems to lie in helping to remove anxiety and making initial encounters with the foreign language and culture as stress-free as possible. But as stated above, when it comes to developing specific linguistic skills, it would appear that captions and subtitles have more benefits to offer if the learner is already at least at intermediate, or better still, advanced level.

3. International subtitling research findings

Over the last two or three decades, a considerable body of research has investigated the question of whether and/or how and to what extent, both captioned and subtitled material can be used for the purposes of foreign, and less frequently, first language learning and development. Most of the studies are so different from one another that they cannot be considered comparable. Studies looking at the value of both subtitles and captions reported upon in the literature have been conducted in a number of different countries and continents with widely divergent subject groups, both in terms of size, age and linguistic capabilities, language pairs etc. For example, taking a case from the early period of research in this field, Danan's work in 1992 involved English speaking university students of French in the USA who were exposed to both captions and subtitles in a university setting. Much more recently, research on captioning in India has been conducted by Kothari et al. (2002) who have studied the contribution of captioned film song and music videos to the development of reading skills of disadvantaged children who watch television for entertainment. Despite the huge range of variables in the various studies conducted to date, fairly consistent findings have emerged.

As it would not be realistic to attempt to provide here a comprehensive review of the studies conducted, a short overview of some of the most frequently cited studies will suffice to provide a context for the discussion of captions and subtitles in minority language contexts which will follow. Going back to the beginning of the period under consideration, research carried out in the 1980s in Canada with young speakers of English and French, who were considered to be "functional bilinguals", involved once-off exposure to nine kinds of input including standard and reversed subtitles and bi-modal input (Lambert et al., 1981). The findings indicated that bi-modal foreign language input and reversed subtitles were much more effective than standard subtitles and other kinds of input in relation to visual/auditory reinforcement.

Two years later, an extensive USA study (Price, 1983) involving 500 students with different native language backgrounds found clear evidence of improved English video comprehension when bi-modal English language input was provided by means of closed captions. Canadian research following up on the 1981 study confirmed the earlier results and tracked improved general comprehension, contextual understanding of concepts, phraseology recall and accuracy of spelling when bi-modal and reversed subtitling were used (Holobow et al., 1984). Similarly, reversed subtitling proved most productive in the 1992 investigation conducted at Michigan Technological University and mentioned above (Danan, 1992). Students of French at beginners and intermediate levels were tested for vocabulary recall by means of cloze tests after having viewed short clips. Bi-modal exposure was also found to produce positive results.

Another study conducted in the same decade in Canada, demonstrated how untranslated audiovisual material can improve auditory processing through its positive impact on motivation, attention and general interest levels (Baltova, 1994). However, the study, which involved intermediate level school pupils of a core French programme, came out clearly in favour of using audiovisual video material in combination with captions and reversed subtitles for maximum effect (ibid.: 516). A later study by the same researcher looked more closely at the advantages to be gained by using specifically bi-modal input (Baltova, 1999). Fast forwarding to more recent research, another study by Danan published in 2004 indicates that both captioning and subtitles are helpful in improving comprehension skills, with subtitles offering "additional cognitive benefits such as greater depth of processing" (Danan, 2004: 67). An important finding was that subtitling can prove more advantageous if language learners are trained to develop active viewing strategies. In other words, informal language learning can be enhanced as a result of more formal pedagogical interventions. Danan (ibid.) also found that new developments in multimedia further augment language learning possibilities. This is due to the fact that learners can now control access to captions and subtitles, enabling them to turn closed subtitles and captions on and off, switch between standard and reversed subtitles, when available, and go back over material.

At Heriot-Watt University in Edinburgh, Vanderplank (1988, 1990, 1993, 1994) carried out a series of studies illustrating the potential for the effective use of captioned teletext audiovisual material to assist intermediate and advanced adult students of English as a second language. Similarly positive findings in relation to reading skills and listening comprehension were also reported during the 1990s in the USA in relation to captions/bimodal input (Neuman and Koskinen, 1990, 1992; Garza, 1991; Borrás and Lafayette, 1994). Very recent research from the Netherlands has provided interesting evidence that young adult Dutch advanced language learners of English can adapt better to regional accents (in this instance, Australian and Scottish) in audiovisual material if they avail of captions rather than standard subtitles to help them (Mitterer and McQueen, 2009).

All in all, the bulk of evidence published to date from the West suggests that captions can only be of very limited assistance to beginner language learners and for that to happen, considerable care must be taken in the selection of suitable material. Indeed Danan (2004: 70) in her review of research on captioning comes to the rather cautious conclusion that "massive exposure to authentic audiovisual material which has not been carefully enough selected or made accessible to non-native viewers can be a very inefficient pedagogical approach". Not surprisingly, most studies confirm that it is mainly at intermediate and advanced levels that captions prove to be most beneficial for foreign language learners.

However, when considering these findings, it must be remembered that they are based to a large extent on research relating to speakers and learners of English and other European languages, who were participating in formal language tuition. The Indian research mentioned above introduces fresh perspectives on how captions can result in more positive outcomes than suggested by Danan, for example, because it investigates how reading captions can help native speakers, rather than foreign language learners, to develop their linguistic skills in informal settings. Kothari (1998, 1999, 2000) and Kothari et al. (2000, 2002) conducted their studies in a very different linguistic environment from those which prevail in North America and Europe. India is a country with a population of 860 million people, only 65 per cent of whom are literate. With 24 official languages and numerous other dialects, the task of improving literacy amongst the remaining 300 million people is an enormous and costly one. It is in this context that the use of captions (called same language subtitling, SLS, in the literature) to improve reading skills has emerged as a practical success with enormous potential. For example, Kothari et al. (2002) demonstrated by means of a controlled experiment that disadvantaged Indian schoolchildren significantly improved their reading skills as a result of watching film songs and music videos with captions. Since "song videos are watched with great passion all over India, in every state and major language", there is enormous scope for the use of captions as a "simple and economical approach to mass literacy skill development in India" (ibid.: 55).

Clearly, in this instance, factors such as the exact correspondence between soundtrack and karaoke-type texts of the song lyrics, as well as the likelihood of regular repetition of the same songs over and over again, contribute significantly to improvements in basic literacy. In addition, the fact that songs are usually viewed in an informal, domestic environment contributes greatly to a positive affective response to learning of this kind amongst the general public. Feedback received from viewers in Gujarat shows that parents are becoming aware of positive secondary, indirect effects of the popularity of the song captions. A parent cited in the article is gratified to see that his young son in Grade 1 always tries to read the captions and as a result, his general interest in reading has increased (ibid.: 64). This Indian research provides concrete evidence that positive first language learning outcomes can result from the use of captions even by children in casual or informal settings: "They will learn a lot because they already like to sing Gujarati songs. They just don't know how the words are written" (ibid.).

As we have seen, on balance studies conducted to date have found that learners at intermediate and advanced level are more likely to make significant linguistic progress as a result of the use of audiovisual material with captions or reversed subtitles, whether in informal or classroom settings. Research has been conducted over many years at the University of Leuven (d'Ydewalle and Pavakanun, 1997; Van de Poel and d'Ydewalle, 1999), into what actually happens when standard subtitles are accessed and processed. This has contributed to a better understanding of what McLoughlin (2009:

175) describes as a complex "process of dynamic association of verbal and non-verbal representation". The researchers have revealed much about how subtitles work by drawing more attention to the complex cognitive processing involved in viewing a film or television programme with the soundtrack in one language while reading subtitles in another. It is now thought that the considerable effort involved in such processing may explain the enhanced recall demonstrated by viewers of subtitled material. Many people are only too familiar with the experience of viewing a foreign film in a language they know with subtitles in their own language. They very quickly realize how difficult it is to avoid reading the subtitles and find it hard to focus completely on the foreign dialogue, even though that is what they would like to do. Indeed, the Leuven research confirms that this is because it is almost impossible to avoid reading subtitles: "Subtitles are not only read mandatorily, but also processed in detail and remembered well" (Van de Poel and d'Ydewalle, 1999: 260).

This ties in with a common criticism, from a language learning perspective, of standard subtitles: that they distract attention from the foreign language soundtrack (Díaz-Cintas and Fernández Cruz, 2008). d'Ydewalle and Gielen (1992) show that this is not necessarily so and that language learners engage with both the soundtrack and subtitles to varying degrees, depending on their foreign language ability and comprehension needs. Where comprehension proved difficult, the viewers were observed to spend more time reading subtitles. The full picture, however, is far from clear. In d'Ydewalle and De Bruycker (2007), a study involving Dutch children and adults, a more regular reading pattern was identified when standard subtitles were provided while reversed subtitles tended to be used intermittently and were sometimes skipped. In general, less time was spent on them and as a result, there were fewer shifts back and forth between the image with the Dutch soundtrack and the English reversed subtitles. Importantly, this study seems to contradict earlier findings elsewhere as it suggests that these learners acquire and retain relatively little of the foreign language used in the reversed subtitles. However, they point out that their research has collected:

a considerable amount of data suggesting that [...] incidental reading of the subtitles in the mother language and hearing the voices in a foreign language, greatly contributes in the incidental acquisition "*of the foreign language vocabulary ... but not of its grammar*". (ibid.: 204, my italics)

Nevertheless, the case for possible beneficial effects of reversed subtitles continues to be argued by scholars, including Kothari et al. (2004), who suggest that having the soundtrack in the viewer's first language allows more time to process the reversed subtitles in the foreign language.

Whatever the relative merits of captions and standard and reversed subtitles, it must be remembered that the very fact that learners at least have the option of making greater or lesser use of written aids when available, has positive effects in terms of greatly reducing the sense of anxiety and nervousness experienced when viewing foreign language audiovisual material, as Vanderplank (1988) has shown. By helping learners to cope with language they do not yet feel comfortable with, subtitles keep them engaged in the language learning process and reduce the risk of frustration, disillusionment and possible complete withdrawal (ibid.). This applies particularly to informal viewing. Recognizing this positive contribution that subtitles can make when students might otherwise feel disheartened, Talaván Zanón (2006) argues that it is important that language teachers use formal situations to point out useful ways in which subtitles can act as a comprehension aid if needed, rather than leaving students to their own devices and risking them developing much feared general over-dependence on subtitles. In short, "students through different training activities, must learn to use subtitles for a reason, other than simply to understand 'everything' that is being said" (ibid.: 43). However, in order for language learners to use subtitles for a reason, it is important for them to have easy and widespread access to them. Unfortunately, this is less frequently the case when it comes to minority languages.

4. Subtitles and minority languages

Returning to the contribution of song captions, Kothari (2002: 64) points
out that captions can be very "covertly educational", while adding to the
overall entertainment value of the viewing experience. Captioned song
lyrics are identified as having specific advantages not offered by ordinary
dialogue captions. For one thing there is, by definition, great interest in
popular song lyrics, it is possible to anticipate some song lyrics, and the
repetition of words, phrases and lines is common. Moreover, songs with
different tempos present "reading challenges for the whole range of literacy
levels" (ibid.). Further advantages include the possibility of reaching a very
large and diverse audience including school-going children, who get reading
reinforcement by watching television in the home environment and adults
with poor literacy, who lack the personal motivation and/or opportunity
to engage in regular reading practice and so make progress.

It is a long way from the 240 languages of India to the scenario in
Ireland where the tiny minority language, Irish, co-exists side by side with
the world's most powerful language, English. But the Indian research cited
above, and the North American and European studies reviewed, do suggest
that untapped audiovisual resources could be more successfully exploited
by those from smaller language communities (d'Ydewalle and De Bruycker,
2007), and also by those interested in the maintenance and development
of minority languages, such as Irish.

In order to illustrate the potential uses of captions and subtitles,
some background information on the Irish language situation is required.
Although Irish and English are the two official languages of the Republic
of Ireland (Éire), the majority of the country's population is Anglophone
with only a limited knowledge of Irish, generally acquired through the primary and secondary school system. The total population is approximately
4.5 million and the number of native speakers of Irish, though continu-
ally contested due to a lack of accurate data, is probably not much more
than 100,000, all of whom also have a command of English. Another 1.5
million can speak Irish with varying degrees of fluency. The language is a

compulsory primary and secondary school subject but many young people leave school having studied Irish for 12 years with much better linguistic skills in French, German or Spanish, for example, which they have probably only studied for 4–5 years. There are many possible explanations for this, some of which relate to the fact that Irish is a minority language. One issue is that being a language used only by a dwindling minority, negative attitudes developed because Irish, like so many other minority languages, became, in the past, associated with backwardness, poverty and remote rural locations and lifestyles. Furthermore, insufficient investment over decades in suitable Irish language teaching methods, textbooks, dictionaries and audiovisual resources took their toll on the learning experience, classroom morale and public attitudes. The fact that Irish is a Celtic language, i.e. a relatively distant relative of the Germanic language, English, has meant that native speakers of English learning Irish have found their first encounters with some typical features somewhat challenging, e.g. Irish typically adopts Verb-Subject-Object word order, has no single word for "yes" and "no", puts nouns into the genitive case after the gerund, has two genders and five declensions, has many more phonemes, including diphthongs than English as spoken in Ireland etc. Finally, like many minority languages, although Irish has a healthy past and contemporary written literature, it is now primarily an oral language strongly rooted in the three main regional variations usually referred to as the Ulster, Connaught and Munster dialects.

The official standard form of Irish has only really been successfully adopted for written purposes but has not had much influence on regional spoken varieties of Irish. So it is that while Irish language television and to a lesser extent, Irish language radio, broadly adhere to the written standard when broadcasting news items and official statements (which originate in a written form), most other material is rooted in one or other of the regional dialects. Native speakers, while comfortable in their own dialect, are not necessarily at ease with the other dialects or when reading the written standard. This is a typical phenomenon in relation to minority languages. Moreover, many native speakers have much higher literacy standards in English than in Irish. This may be due in part to schooling and level of education and also to the relative dearth of Irish language newspapers, magazines and popular literature. In short, Irish faces many challenges which are typical of minority languages and many of which may be addressed, at least in a partial way, by the judicious use of captions and/or subtitles. The challenges include (a) difficulties which arise as a result of relatively small number of native speakers, (b) the proximity of a much stronger linguistic neighbour, (c) the restriction of everyday use to limited, often social and/or domestic domains, (d) the relative weakness of the standard written form in relation to regional oral varieties, (e) the lack of an agreed widely implemented spoken standard, and (f) limited specialized terminology and problems with terminological dissemination and uptake, amongst others.

The field of language planning and policy are concerned with positive interventions which can be made to support a minority language with this sort of problems (O'Connell and Walsh, 2006: 22–34). Status planning (granting official recognition), corpus planning (creating new forms and terminology) and acquisition planning (teaching and learning the language) are all key concepts in this context. When Irish became the first official language of the State, in 1937, it was a major boost at the level of status. But the harsh economic reality of poverty in and emigration from Irish speaking areas (known as An Ghaeltacht), up to the 1970s and 1980s did a lot to undermine the language. In recent years, some major progress has occurred at the level of status. This includes the establishment, in 1996, of the country's first and only Irish language television station, originally called TnaG, but renamed TG4 in 1996. This media initiative has been very positive as far as prestige and positive image creation is concerned and in practical terms too because it provides a minimum of six hours of daily core programming in Irish. Television is a particularly prestigious audiovisual medium for a minority language, not least because minority languages are so often traditionally associated with backwardness. There can be little doubt that the arrival and success of TG4 has helped to reverse negative attitudes and stereotypes which have dogged Irish for decades. Moreover, since Gaeltacht communities are geographically distant, television provides a way of forging a new, virtual linguistic community, linking Irish speaking homes both inside and outside An Ghaeltacht and across political borders between the Republic of Ireland and Northern Ireland, which is part of the UK, and even further afield, thanks to satellite technology.

Corpus planning too is of critical importance for minority languages which are always under pressure due to lack of resources and native speakers to create and disseminate new terminology. Terminology work can be slow and expensive, especially if there is considerable dependence on the use of hardcopy, e.g. glossaries, dictionaries, textbooks. Fortunately, the internet has recently opened up wonderful, cost effective alternatives in this regard. And now, Irish language television can offer new and very immediate informal ways to allow speakers and learners to encounter the new vocabulary, which is vital if the language is to facilitate communication in the twenty-first century. Irish language television also has some positive implications for acquisition planning because intergeneration transmission (the traditional way in which both major and minority languages are passed on), has been greatly weakened as a result of the fact that children now often live far away from their grandparents and other Irish speaking relatives. Television offers the hope that in the comfort of their own homes and in a relaxed informal environment, speakers and learners of Irish can develop certain linguistic skills from listening to television characters, rather than members of the extended family, as in the past.

Until relatively recently in Ireland, subtitles in cinema were rare and more or less limited to European art house productions shown at film clubs. Subtitles on television are also a relatively new phenomenon and one largely associated with English television for SDH, on the one hand, and with standard subtitles in English used widely in the case of minority language broadcasting in Irish, on the other. As far as interlingual subtitles are concerned, in recent decades, the national broadcasters, RTE and TG4, have tended to use these almost exclusively in one direction and for one purpose, i.e. English subtitles to render Irish language programmes intelligible to those with little or no understanding of Irish. Largely for financial and pragmatic reasons, both Irish captions on Irish language programmes and Irish subtitles on English language programmes are very rare, despite the fact that many sound pedagogical arguments could be made in favour of introducing them. It is likely that neither minority broadcasting policy makers nor educationalists fully appreciate the contribution that informal learning through television could make to the future of this and other minority languages and that general attitudes still reflect the old association of language skills development primarily with formal learning situations.

The rationale for the current subtitling status quo in Ireland whereby Irish programmes have English subtitles but not vice versa, and English programmes have SDH captions but Irish programmes do not, has much to do with the very real need to win and keep public Anglophone support for Irish language broadcasting funded by the Irish taxpayer but little to do with the potential role of broadcasting in informal and lifelong learning. This is not to attempt to undermine in any way the huge cultural and linguistic achievement of Irish language broadcasting to date, it is, rather, to highlight that there is still much to be done.

Applying the general findings on the benefits of captions and subtitles for language learners to the minority language situation in Ireland, it is clear that the introduction of Irish language subtitles on Irish language programmes (bi-modal Irish input) and on English language programmes (standard subtitles for native speakers of Irish and revered subtitles for English speakers) could have considerable incidental benefits for intermediate and advanced learners of Irish, as well as for native speakers, especially if they do not enjoy high language literacy levels. The latter would gain reading confidence through increased exposure to the standard written form. Moreover, those who are unfamiliar with dialects other than their own would have the crutch of captions to help the development of greater cohesion between disparate regions of native speakers. Referring back to the main challenges faced by minority languages mentioned above, increased exposure to Irish captions and subtitles on national television could counteract to an extent the all pervasive presence of English in the public domain, extend the range of domains in which Irish is spoken daily by disseminating new terminology quickly and efficiently, develop and reinforce the written standard amongst native speakers and learners alike and improve understanding of regional dialects. Furthermore, the existence of a greater volume of Irish captioned and subtitled material would be of obvious benefit in more formal language learning environments as well.

The current practice of broadcasting programmes in Irish with subtitles in English, largely motivated by the need to attract as large a viewing audience as possible and build national goodwill towards Irish, would seem likely to have a gradual adverse effect on the Irish language competence of both native speakers and fluent Irish viewers since the programmes which they watch are not monolingual Irish but a combination of the weaker Irish audio and the stronger visual/written mode reinforcing English. This is a point that needs to receive the serious attention of language planners and educationalists as its effects could be far-reaching over a generation (O'Connell, 1999, 2000).

References

Baltova, I. (1994), The Impact of Video on the Comprehension Skills of Core French Students. *The Canadian Modern Language Review* 50, 507–32.

—— (2000), (1999), Multisensory Language Teaching in a Multidimensional Curriculum: The Use of Authentic Bimodal Video in Core French. *Canadian Modern Language Review* 56(1), 32–48.

Borrás, I., and R. Lafayette (1994), Effects of Multimedia Courseware Subtitling on the Speaking Performance of College Students of French. *The Modern Language Journal* 78(1), 61–75.

Danan, M. (1992) Reversed Subtitling and Dual Coding Theory: New Directions for Foreign Language Instruction. *Language Learning* 42(4), 497–527.

—— (2004), Captioning and Subtitling: Undervalued Language Learning Strategies. *Meta* 49(1), 67–77.

De Bruycker, W., and G. d'Ydewalle (2003), Reading Native and Foreign Language Television Subtitles in Children and Adults. In J. Hyona, R. Radach and H. Deubel (eds), *The Mind's Eye: Cognitive and Applied Aspects of Eye Movement Research*. Amsterdam: Elsevier Science BV, 671–84.

d'Ydewalle, G., and W. De Bruycker (2007), Eye Movements of Children and Adults While Reading Television Subtitles. *European Psychologist* 12(3), 96–205.

d'Ydewalle, G., and I. Gielen (1992), Attention Allocation with Overlapping Sound, Image, and Text. In K. Rayner (ed.), *Eye Movement and Visual Cognition: Scene Perceptions and Reading*. New York: Springer Verlag, 413–27.

d'Ydewalle G., and U. Pavakanun (1992), Watching Foreign TV Programs and Language Learning. In F. Engel, D. Bouwhuis, T. Bösser and G. d'Ydewalle (eds), *Cognitive Modelling and Interactive Environments in Language Learning.* Berlin: Springer Verlag, 193–8.

d'Ydewalle, G., and U. Pavakanun (1997), Could Enjoying a Movie Lead to Language Acquisition? In P. Winterhoff and T. Van der Voort (eds), *New Horizons in Media Psychology.* Opladen (FRG): Westdeutscher Verlag, 145–55.

d'Ydewalle, G., J. Van Rensbergen and J. Pollet (1987), Reading a Message When the Same Message is Available Auditorily in Another Language: The Case of Subtitling. In J. K. O'Regan and A. Levy-Schoen (eds), *Eye Movements: From Physiology to Cognition.* Amsterdam: North-Holland, 313–21.

Díaz-Cintas, J., and M. Fernández Cruz (2008), Using Subtitled Material for Foreign Language Instruction. In J. Díaz-Cintas (ed.), *The Didactics of Audiovisual Translation.* Amsterdam: John Benjamins, 201–14.

Garza, T. J. (1991), Evaluating the Use of Captioned Video Materials in Advanced Foreign Language Learning. *Foreign Language Annals* 24(3), 239–58.

Holobow, N. E., W. E. Lambert and L. Sayegh (1984), Pairing Script and Dialog: Combinations that Show Promise for Second or Foreign Language Learning. *Language Learning* 34, 59–76.

Koolstra, C. M., and J. W. J. Beentjes (1999), Children's Vocabulary Acquisition in a Foreign Language Through Watching Subtitled Television Programs at Home. *Educational Technology* 47(1), 51–60.

Kothari, B. (1999), Same-Language Subtitling: Integrating Post Literacy Development and Popular Culture on Television, *Media and Technology for Human Resource Development* 11(3), 111–17.

—— (2000), Same-Language Subtitling on Indian Television: Harnessing the Power of Popular Culture for Literacy. In K. Wilkins (ed.), *Redeveloping Communication for Social Change: Theory, Practice and Power.* New York: Rowman and Littlefield, 135–46.

——, A. Pandey and A. R. Chudgar (2004), Reading Out of The Idiot Box: Same-Language Subtitling on TV in India. *Information Technologies and International Development* 2(1), 23–44.

——, J. Takeda, A. Joshi and A. Pandey (2002), Same-Language Subtitling: A Butterfly for Literacy? *International Journal of Lifelong Education* 21(1), 55–66.

Lambert, W. E., I. Boehler and N. Sidoti (1981), Choosing the Languages of Subtitles and Spoken Dialogs for Media Presentations: Implications for Second Language Acquisition. *Applied Psycholinguistics* 2, 133–48.

McLoughlin, L. (2009), Subtitles in Translators' Training: A Model of Analysis. *Romance Studies* 27(3), 174–85.

Mitterer, H., and J. M. McQueen (2009), Foreign Subtitles Help but Native-Language Subtitles Harm Foreign Speech Perception. *PLoS ONE* 4(11): e7785. Available from: <http://www.plosone.org/article/info:doi/10.1371/journal. pone.0007785> (accessed 08/07/2010).

Neuman, S., and P. Koskinen (1990), *Using Captioned Television to Improve the Reading Proficiency of Language Minority Students.* Falls Church, VA, USA: National Captioning Institute.

—— (1992), Captioned Television as Comprehensible Input: Effects of Incidental Language Learning from Contexts for Language Minority Students. *Reading Research Quarterly* 27, 95–106.

O'Connell, E. (1999), Subtitles on Screen: Something for Everyone in the Audience? *Teanga* 18, 85–91.

—— (2000), The Role of Screen Translation: A Response. In H. Kelly-Holmes (ed.), *Current Issues in Language and Society (Minority Language Broadcasting – Breton and Irish)* 7(2), 169–74.

O'Connell, E. and J. Walsh (2006), The Translation Boom: Irish and Language Planning in the 21st Century. *Administration, the Journal of the IPA* 54(3), 22–43.

Price, K. (1983), Closed-Captioned TV: An Untapped Resource. *MATSOL Newsletter* 12, 7–8.

Talaván Zanón, N. (2006), Using Subtitles to Enhance Foreign Language Learning. *Porta Linguarum* 6, 41–52.

van de Poel, M., and G. d'Ydewalle (1999), Incidental Foreign-Language Acquisition by Children while Watching Subtitled Television Programs. In Y. Gambier and H. Gottlieb (eds), *(Multi)Media Translation: Concepts, Practices and Research.* Amsterdam: John Benjamin, 259–74.

Vanderplank, R. (1988), The Value of Teletext Subtitles in Language Learning. *English Language Teaching (ELT) Journal* 42(4), 272–81.

—— (1990), Paying Attention to the Words: Practical and Theoretical Problems in Watching TV Programmes with Unilingual (Ceefax) Subtitles. *System* 18(2), 221–34.

—— (1993), A Very Verbal Medium: Language Learning Through Closed Captions. *TESOL Journal* 3(1), 10–14.

—— (1994), Resolving Inherent Conflicts: Autonomous Language Learning from Popular Broadcast Television. In H. Jung and R. Vanderplank (eds), *Barriers and Bridges: Media Technology in Language Learning,* Proceedings of the 1993 CETaLL Symposium on the Occasion of the 10th AILA World Congress. Frankfurt: Peter Lang, 119–34.

ELISA PEREGO AND ELISA GHIA

Subtitle Consumption according to Eye Tracking Data: An Acquisitional Perspective

1. Introduction

Since its very first inception back in the 1960s, eye tracking technology has been widely exploited to study the overall mechanisms of the human visual system in a number of different areas. These include, for instance, marketing and medical research, product design, human-computer interaction, perceptual psychology, psycholinguistics and cognitive linguistics. In recent years, eye tracking has entered the field of translation studies (Göpferich et al., 2008) and has started to be exploited in relation to audiovisual translation (AVT) to investigate the processing of audiovisual input (Reichle et al., 2007; Smith, 2004). Scholars researching in this field became very much aware that knowing more about user perception might offer the necessary tools to produce more successful translations. In this chapter, we will focus on eye tracking employed to explore the visual attention and the reading behaviour of audiences exposed to captions and subtitles,[1] even though its use in the field of AVT may go far beyond that.

The need to resort to eye tracking when studying AVT is strictly linked to the increasingly important issues of usability and accessibility to the media for both unimpaired audiences and viewers with sensory impairment (Díaz-Cintas and Anderman, 2009). Viewers who access a subtitled product necessarily deal with a composite text and are required to decipher

---

1 Typically, subtitles are the translation of the source dialogue while captions are the transcription of the dialogue in the same language as the original soundtrack and they are designed for the hearing impaired.

a whole set of semiotic channels. Given the crucial role of captions and subtitles in supporting viewers with or without special needs, and since subtitles are an added overlay in a semiotically intricate aggregate, one of the main purposes of subtitling companies and of subtitlers should be to ensure accessibility and to maximize usability. On the one hand, the foundation of accessibility is to offer viewers equal opportunity to access the service and use it regardless of potential disabilities. In terms of perceptual characteristics of the text, this is obtained, for example, by implementing readability, or by making subtitles for the deaf or for second language learners constantly available as an option. On the other hand, usability is meant to offer easy to use, satisfying and user-oriented products which are cognitively effective and processed effortlessly. Usability is obtained, for instance, by implementing readability.

Readability is intended as the "quality that makes possible the recognition of the information content of material when it is represented by alphanumeric characters in meaningful groupings, such as words, sentences, or continuous text", while legibility pertains to "the attribute of alphanumeric characters that makes it possible for each one to be identifiable from others" (Sanders and McCormick, 1993: 121). The two terms are often confused and used interchangeably. However, the former refers to the ease of reading as determined by the organization of information units and by typographic design as a whole; the latter refers to the ease with which a person manages to identify characters or letters.

Nowadays, legibility (i.e. the degree to which printed information on screen is unambiguous and distinguishable based on appearance) is no longer an issue. Refined modern equipment and sophisticated techniques used to generate subtitles often secure the quality of both definition and discernability of characters on screen. Securing readability (i.e. the degree at which printed information on screen is unambiguous on the basis of language fluency, content and meaning, quantity of text delivered, and message communicated), however, is a far more difficult task. Reading ease can result from the combination of content delivered, style used, and design or text structure chosen. So, "even a legible typeface can become unreadable through poor setting and placement, just as a less legible typeface can be made more readable through good design" (Craig and Scala, 2006: 63).

In subtitling, for instance, attention is being increasingly drawn to technical, positional and aesthetic criteria. The interest in improving subtitle ease of use and efficiency of processing, especially via careful text display and formatting, is to be ascribed to the ever increasing acknowledgement of the utility of subtitles for second language learning purposes (Díaz-Cintas and Fernández Cruz, 2008), to assist the development of literacy (Kothari, 2000), and to the firm rooting and rapid growth of practices, such as captioning for deaf and hard of hearing viewers, which are meant for an audience who deserves impeccable usability standards (Díaz-Cintas et al., 2007).

Linguistic and translational aspects of subtitling are no less important in a usability-oriented perspective. Various methods have been devised and adopted to find the closest formal and semantic correspondents in the target language whilst reducing the source text (ST) and converting it from spoken to written mode. The literature and the bibliographical repertoires available show the escalating interest in this area (Ivarsson, 2009). As a matter of fact, nowadays well-established translational strategies exist and are followed by most subtitlers. Little experimental research, however, has been carried out to shed light on the way such strategies impact on viewers, or on their role in enhancing or limiting the usability of a translated text. In the same vein, when it comes to structural criteria, hardly any have been tested empirically in spite of their importance.

Eye tracking research in subtitling has started to shed light on several issues concerning overall subtitle consumption. In what follows, a concise overview of the most significant results is provided, along with a more detailed description of two case studies conducted recently. The former focuses on the way certain qualitative and translational aspects of subtitles can impact on second language learners (Ghia, forthcoming). The latter concentrates on the effect of high vs. low quality line segmentation on subtitle reading and comprehension (Perego et al., 2010). The focus of the discussion eventually moves specifically into the area of second language acquisition.

2. Eye tracking results on subtitle consumption

For starters, one of the earliest and most interesting eye tracking based results regards the automaticity hypothesis, whereby viewers show a strong tendency to read subtitles at their onset (d'Ydewalle and De Bruycker, 2007; d'Ydewalle and Gielen, 1992). Attention to subtitles seems to occur independently of both viewer- and input-specific variables. Viewers appear to read subtitles no matter what their sex and age are (d'Ydewalle et al., 1989), regardless of any hearing impairment (Verfaillie and d'Ydewalle, 1987), and independently of their familiarity with watching subtitled films in general (d'Ydewalle and Gielen, 1992; d'Ydewalle et al., 1991; Ghia, forthcoming).

Furthermore, concurrent attention to soundtrack and visuals is not impeded by subtitle reading: viewers are able to attend to auditory and visual stimuli simultaneously and effectively (d'Ydewalle and De Bruycker, 2007; d'Ydewalle and Gielen, 1992; Perego et al., 2010), with visuals seemingly facilitating subtitle understanding – and, in general, the processing of any media communicated message – especially when they provide an appropriate context to the viewer (Grimes, 1991; Lang, 2001; Perego et al., 2010).

As far as input-specific factors are concerned, not even soundtrack availability, scene characteristics and audiovisual genre, for instance, appear to prevent viewers from reading subtitles. Subtitle reading has been shown to occur in both the presence and the absence of concurrent spoken dialogue in the auditory dimension, and independently of viewers' mastery of the language heard in it (d'Ydewalle et al., 1987). Similarly, audiovisual genre and scene integration with dialogue do not hinder overall attention to the subtitles. All of these input-specific factors, however, were found to affect reading times and general viewing patterns (de Linde and Kay, 1999; d'Ydewalle and Gielen, 1992). In a study focused on audiovisual genre, viewers were observed to read the subtitles when exposed to both films and news broadcasts. With news broadcasts, however, longer reading times and earlier and faster shifts from the visuals to the written text were recorded. This trend was attributed to the greater density of information that subtitles contain in news as compared to films, and to the overall faster pace of news broadcasts, which caused viewers to shift more quickly to the subtitle area and spend more time on it (d'Ydewalle and Gielen, 1992). In cognitive terms, these findings can relate to the greater complexity required in the processing of news broadcasts as compared to films, which can be ascribed to a lower degree of audio-video redundancy typically operating in this genre.

Although not impeding subtitle reading, processing complexity can be likewise associated with subtitle relation to the characteristics of shots and scenes. In an intralingual subtitling condition, for instance, it was found that shot changes across subtitles and subtitle reference to off-screen rather than on-screen speakers resulted in increased re-reading of the subtitles and a growth in deflections, i.e. vertical shifts from the images to the subtitles (de Linde and Kay, 1999: 72–3). Even in this case, the intensified visual activity is interpretable as the result of a greater processing effort, associated with conditions of incongruence between scenes and subtitles.

A similar effect is triggered by certain linguistic features in interlingual subtitles, where word frequency and lexical cohesion are liable to affect fixation duration and reading time. A recent study by Moran (2008) showed that reading times on the subtitle area tended to decrease if subtitles contained high-frequency words or repeated words (vs. pro-forms). Longer and more explicit subtitles seemed therefore to be more readable and usable than standard length subtitles, and they seemed to ensure easier processing and better comprehension of the target text (TT).[2]

In addition to those listed so far, other input-specific factors, such as subtitle translation and subtitle layout, have been proven to affect subtitle consumption. On the one hand, the effect of different types of translation has been explored in the context of interlingual subtitling meant for different audiences. In particular, research drawing on eye tracking

2   Interestingly, this contradicts most of the traditional literature on subtitling, which claims that a reduced translation is a necessary condition enabling viewers to process subtitles effectively (Ivarsson and Carroll, 1998; Smith, 1998).

methodology has specifically taken into account how new, nonconventional subtitling strategies impact on general audiences (Caffrey, 2008a, 2008b) and how certain conventional subtitling strategies (i.e. formal simplification vs. literal transfer) impact on language learners (namely users exploiting subtitled audiovisual input as a tool for learning foreign languages) (Ghia, forthcoming). On the other hand, empirically grounded experiments have been conducted to detect how differently segmented two-line subtitles impact on viewers (Perego et al., 2010). In the following paragraphs a brief overview of the above-mentioned case studies is provided.

3. The effect of translation strategies on subtitle consumption

Fansubbed *anime* are Japanese animations purposefully subtitled by fans for fans and made freely available on the net. A cognitively taxing situation has been observed when consuming fansubbed *anime*, which is caused by the nature of the product itself. Fansubs are a typical case of abusive experimental subtitling, characterized by "thick" and overexplicitating translations (Appiah, 2000) proved to be overloading to viewers, no matter how interested they are in the product. The extent of the taxing effect of specific features of fansubs (e.g. the presence of pop-up glosses, i.e. notes that frequently come out on screen to explain culturally marked items) has been successfully detected thanks to a thorough analysis of eye tracking data comprising saccade-based, fixation-based and pupillometric measurements as variables enabling to appraise viewers' processing effort (Caffrey, 2008a, 2008b).

In a recent study by Ghia (forthcoming), the use of eye tracking methods proved to be useful also in exploring the mapping processes inherent to the reception of differently subtitled audiovisual texts by L2 learners – by mapping implying the comparison which tends to be systematically operated between the ST and the TT when simultaneously accessed. The study involved monitoring learners' visual activity during exposure to subtitled audiovisual input featuring the use of different translation strategies in the subtitles. The strategies in question were divided into a general condition of literalness and equivalence of form, operating at the lexical and syntactic level (Examples 1 and 3), and one of greater divergence between ST and TT. Divergence was either quantitative, as achieved through the use of formal simplification (Example 5), or rather qualitative, as resulting from the substitution of lexical items (Example 2) and syntactic-pragmatic patterns from the ST with formally non-equivalent patterns in the TT (Example 4). Substitution involved the use of semantically distinct lexical items or the exploitation of different syntactic structures, often implying concurrent variations in the pragmatic value of the utterance. One common instance of the latter situation was the substitution of questioning structures in the ST with imperatives in the TT, affecting not only the sentence syntax, but also its pragmatic connotation (Example 3).

Example 1. Formal equivalence at the lexical level

English ST: *And what happens next in the dream?*
Italian TT: *E cosa succede poi nel sogno?*
Back translation: And what happens next in the dream?

Example 2. Lexical substitution (qualitative divergence)

English ST: *And what happens next in the dream?*
Italian TT: *E cosa succede poi nella favola?*
Back translation: And what happens next in the fable?

Example 3. Formal equivalence at the syntactic level

English ST: *Mr Thacker, will you come this way?*
Italian TT: *Mr Thacker, vuole venire da questa parte?*
Back-translation: Mr Thacker, will you come this way?

Example 4. Syntactic substitution (qualitative divergence)

English ST: *Mr Thacker, will you come this way?*
Italian TT: *Mr Thacker, venga da questa parte.*
Back translation: Mr Thacker, come this way.

Example 5. Reduction (quantitative divergence)

English ST: Any horses *in that one?*
Italian TT: Qualche cavallo?
Back-translation: Any horses?

The results of the experiment show the occurrence of an intensified visual activity in the presence of diverging translation, as detected through the analysis of both deflections and fixations. A significantly higher amount of deflections was performed in the presence of non-literal as compared to literal translation. The trend was especially manifest when the divergence between ST and TT was qualitative and lexical (lexical substitution, Example 2) or quantitative (reduction, Example 5). Furthermore, most second-pass fixations performed during deflections occurred on diverging content words, and most often involved the re-reading of isolated strings and items rather than entire subtitles.

Along the cognitive dimension, findings indicate a variation in mapping between ST and TT related to the use of different translational strategies. As mentioned above, when exposed to subtitled input learners tend to constantly perform a process of ST-TT mapping (Karamitroglou, 1998). The extent of the mapping operated varies, among other factors, as a function of linguistic proficiency in the L2 and the characteristics of the subtitles. In translational terms, findings indicate that lexical variation from L2 dialogue and omissions of part of it in the L1 subtitles are bound to intensify the extent of mapping performed. Co-occurring growing attention to the verbal dimension is then suggested by the targets of second-pass fixations, which in most cases were recorded to fall on the diverging lexical items themselves.

4. The effect of line segmentation on subtitle consumption

Another input-specific aspect that has been studied via eye tracking is subtitle layout. As mentioned above, aspects of the appearance of subtitles,
i.e. their screen attributes and format, have been cared for since subtitling
started to exist based on the general motto that subtitles have to be invis-
ible to the viewer (Smith, 1998). This means that subtitles should not cor-
rupt the image nor should they distract the audience. Their presentation
should be as unobtrusive as possible from both an aesthetic and a cognitive
point of view.

Most traditional studies on the subject (Díaz-Cintas, 2003; Ivarsson
and Carroll, 1998; Tveit, 2004) tackle the technical aspects of subtitling
starting from the assumption that reading speed is influenced by the manner
in which the text is presented but also by the quantity and complexity of
the information that is conveyed, and by the action on screen at a given
moment. Medium-based constraints relating to time and space do the rest
in imposing most of the technical criteria in subtitling. The space available
on the screen, along with the reading speed of viewers and the amount of
written material they can take in while watching a non-self-paced subtitled
product, have always determined the nature of subtitles and the recourse
to such translation strategies as elimination and condensation. The fact
that the original text needs to be heavily abridged and adjusted for the
above-mentioned reasons determines the number of characters to appear
per line and the number of lines to be featured per subtitle.

Specifically, d'Ydewalle and De Bruycker (2007) concentrated on
the latter point by exploring how subtitle line distribution in interaction
with subtitle language affected general viewing behaviour. The eye movements of both children and adults were monitored whilst watching films
with one-line or two-line subtitles in either standard (L2 dialogue with
L1 titles) or reversed (L1 dialogue with L2 titles) subtitling conditions.
Findings showed an interaction between subtitle language and subtitle
layout, with standard subtitling correlating with more regular reading
patterns in the presence of two-liners, and the reversed condition being

associated with more regular reading in the presence of one-liners. The reversed condition, however, generally entailed more irregular reading patterns, as manifest in the greater occurrence of subtitle skipping, longer latency times (the time gaps occurring between the appearance of a stimulus and the ensuing saccade), and fewer fixations on words in the subtitles. Standard interlingual subtitles spreading over two lines thus appeared to be the condition requiring the least processing effort and favouring the smoothest viewing behaviour.

Medium-specific limitations and technical requirements in subtitling additionally influence further layout factors such as subtitle location, the presentation and alignment of lines, and line segmentation, which comes into play when long subtitles need to be broken down. Besides fulfilling aesthetic and geometric criteria, text distribution and subtitle division are considered central to minimize subtitle intrusion and cognitive load on viewers (Karamitroglou, 1998).

When two-line subtitles have to be used, the way they must be structured in order to boost readability becomes a main concern, especially when having to deal with long sentences. This led scholars to search for the ideal architecture of the subtitled text. Whenever it is not possible to use a single-line self-contained subtitle, the way in which the text is broken into two lines has always been a concern among scholars, though it does not seem to have been an issue for subtitle producers. The stance shared by many scholars on a predominantly intuitive basis has for a long time been that when words are intimately connected by logic, semantics or grammar they should be written on the same line, thus keeping constituents together and breaking subtitles down into "digestible chunks" (Smith, 1998: 118; Díaz-Cintas, 2003; Ivarsson and Carroll, 1998). It has always been taken for granted that matching line breaks with sentence blocks is particularly advisable for special audiences with linguistic or sensory impairments such as immigrants having to acquire or improve literacy in a second language, young children learning to read, deaf and hard of hearing, older adults (Ivarsson and Carroll, 1998; Tveit, 2004). Coherent line segmentation is also considered desirable whenever subtitles are exploited for second language learning purposes, or when the original is very hard to follow (as, for instance, when information density is high, speech rate fast, the quantity of culture-bound items is large, and information conveyed by speech is not redundant with information conveyed by visuals).

Psycholinguistic literature on reading seems to support this idea. Starting from the consideration that normal reading is organized into word groups corresponding to syntactic units, and that its ease and speed in different reading situations seem to be affected by layout (Chaparro et al., 2005; Henderson et al., 1995), it is possible to put forward the hypothesis that an individual's reading ease will be influenced by the way in which lines are segmented (Perego, 2008). The idea is that reading would be more fluent when subtitle editing takes into account constituency and that a coherent segmentation of subtitles spanning over two lines can enhance gist comprehension, word recognition, and scene recognition. On the contrary, a poor, non-coherent segmentation can disrupt the reading flow, thus hindering film comprehension and both word and scene recognition. So, since normal reading is a sequential and holistic process which occurs in chunks (Coltheart, 1987; Rayner and Pollatsek, 1987) and in a partially automatic and effortless way (LaBerge and Samuls, 1974; Perfetti, 1985), such process can be enhanced by subtitles ending at natural linguistic breaks, ideally at clause or phrase boundaries. The idea that subtitles should be divided coherently is so strong that it is also advocated in most literature on the didactics of subtitling: teaching prospective subtitlers to care for text distribution, formatting and segmentation seems to be part of most specialized AVT training curricula (James et al., 1996; Díaz-Cintas, 2003, 2008; Kruger, 2008).

In spite of these recommendations, whether paying attention to this structural aspect when generating captions or subtitles determines the quality of the final outcome remained to be proven until very recently. Whether poor segmentation really causes perceptual confusion and is to be accounted for as a burden on perception and cognitive effectiveness has been tested experimentally in a study taking into account at the same time eye movements, visual scene processing performance, and subtitle processing performance (Perego et al., 2010). The need to establish the impact of subtitle segmentation on film viewers' comprehension and memory rose from the need to shed light, through experimental evidence, on the assumed superiority of a syntactically logical segmentation. Since non-coherent segmentation can easily be avoided, results could give helpful hints on how to treat an aspect of subtitling which could be considered more often, so long as other technical constraints are respected.

Recall that in their work the authors refer to non-coherent, unpredictable and unnaturally segmented subtitles as to "low-quality" or "ill-segmented" subtitles (Example 6); when segmentation follows the basic rules of syntax, the subtitles are referred to as "proficient", "high-quality" or "well-segmented" subtitles (Example 7).

Example 6. Well-segmented subtitle

Cantavamo per i villaggi ungheresi.	We would sing in various Hungarian villages.

Example 7. Ill-segmented subtitle

Cantavamo per i villaggi ungheresi.	We would sing in various Hungarian villages.

The eye tracking experiment on subtitled film processing shows that, contrary to expectations – i.e. ill-segmented subtitles hinder information processing and slow down the reading process (Brondeel, 1994; Ivarsson and Carroll, 1998; James et al., 1996; Karamitroglou, 1998; Kruger, 2008; Perego, 2008; Smith, 1998) –, participants appear to overall process well-segmented and ill-segmented subtitles in the same way and with the same outcomes. Technically, the number of fixations on the visuals and on the subtitled area did not differ significantly in both experimental conditions, nor did the mean fixation duration. This enabled the authors to claim that subtitle segmentation quality does not have such a significant impact over viewers' performance and over their cognitive processing and recognition capacity. If any, a significant – though small – difference was nonetheless detected in the mean fixation duration within the subtitled region, where fixations on ill-segmented subtitles were only slightly longer than fixations on well-segmented subtitles. Furthermore, although the analyses did not show any improvement in general and specific comprehension tests that could be attributed to the quality of subtitling segmentation, researchers obtained a slightly lower gist comprehension when high-quality subtitles were presented in the first part of the movie.

5. Subtitle consumption and second language acquisition

The above overview of eye tracking based findings on subtitle reading and processing provides a picture of how subtitles are typically consumed by viewers. Knowing that, it is possible to extend the reflection onto the way subtitles could be used for acquisitional purposes.

Undeniably, research has long been stressing the potential of subtitled audiovisual input on the learning and maintenance of an L2 and the spreading of literacy, as inspired by reports from so-called subtitling countries (Danan, 2004). Empirical studies have been conducted, and most of them have addressed the acquisition of specific linguistic competencies (e.g. listening and production skills, vocabulary development and syntactic accuracy) in either short-term exposure contexts (Markham and Peter, 2002; Van de Poel and d'Ydewalle, 2001; Van Lommel et al., 2006) or after more prolonged viewing of subtitled audiovisual input over time (Ghia, 2007). Acquisitional studies, however, have rarely been exploiting eye tracking as a resource to shed light on the cognitive processes taking place during the reception of subtitled input by language learners (Ghia, forthcoming). What follows is thus a series of L2 acquisition-oriented reflections emerging from the eye tracking based findings we previously illustrated.

The fact that a strong tendency to read subtitles exists, that subtitles do not overtax viewers and that mapping tends to constantly occur can account for the high incidental learning rate recorded in subtitling countries, and can make subtitled products a precious resource for second language learning to be considered and exploited in typically dubbing areas alike. By providing a translation of L2 speech, subtitles can make comprehensible to learners input which would otherwise be too complex to access, thus fulfilling one fundamental prerequisite to language acquisition, i.e. the availability of comprehensible input in the L2 (Krashen, 1985). The facilitative function of subtitles is directly related to the mapping mechanism between ST and TT inherent to the reception of subtitled input by L2 learners. As mentioned above, a factor affecting the degree of linguistic mapping operated is the level of linguistic proficiency in the L2, with beginning learners tending to focus on isolated lexical items and more advanced learners to shift to more elaborate and critical processing at the syntactic and pragmatic level (Nobili, 1995). Whereas subtitles may assist less proficient learners in the decoding of short chunks in the L2, they may in parallel foster a more holistic reflection on general linguistic usage in the foreign language among more advanced learners.

Specific features of subtitles in terms of their layout and linguistic-translational characteristics could additionally impact on L2 learning. As previously summarized, research has mainly concentrated on the perception of subtitles varying in overall cohesion among each other and the frequency of the words contained in them (Moran, 2008), their translation (Ghia, forthcoming), and their distribution and segmentation across lines (d'Ydewalle and De Brucyker, 2007; Perego et al., 2010).[3]

Along an acquisitional perspective, subtitles showing explicit cohesive ties to each other might assist learners in the overall comprehension of the audiovisual text, enabling them to retrieve information more easily and avoid ambiguity of reference. In parallel, the presence of high-frequency words in the subtitles might also reveal beneficial to language learners, since it accelerates reading and can potentially leave more attentional resources available for the decoding of the dialogic dimension and the intake of meaningfully contextualized L2 input.

---

3   The degree of dialogue contextualization within scenes is yet another feature of audiovisual input likely to have an impact on L2 learning. Space limitations and the focus of the present contribution, however, do not make it possible to deal with the issue in detail.

Subtitle translation can similarly have an impact on foreign language acquisition. Ghia's (forthcoming) experimental study showed that formal non-equivalence between ST and TT resulted in the increased performance of deflections by L2 learners, as well as in the repeated fixation of the diverging items in the subtitles. In processing terms, the observed trend may be attributed to the growing allocation of attention to the diverging items, and the occurrence of intensified mapping between ST and TT in the presence of a high translational divergence between them. The phenomena, in turn, document overall greater focus on the verbal component of input (Tanenhaus, 2007).

One possible cognitive explanation of the trend could lie in the fact that a diverging TT translation creates a disruption in the reception of input, resulting in more attentive processing and enhanced focus on specific linguistic components. In perceptual terms, the process is one of perceptual salience, which by definition stems from a "surprise effect" and a deviation from most likely expectations about input (Smith, 2004). In our case, it stems from expectations about close translational correspondence between ST and TT. Along the acquisitional perspective, the phenomenon is the basis for input enhancement, with reference to the whole set of input manipulations aimed at increasing the perceptual salience of input components and at shifting learners' attention to them, thus potentially paving the way for learning (Sharwood-Smith, 1993). Different translation strategies can thus be suitable for language learning, even though they cognitively operate in the opposite direction: on the one hand, the easification and acceleration of processing by literal rendering of dialogue facilitate the matching of ST and TT items; on the other hand, the complexification of dialogue-subtitle mapping by means of formal simplification or substitution of patterns across translation may promote deeper processing and more refined analysis of input, which are in turn believed to be facilitative of language acquisition.

Similar considerations can ensue from findings concerning subtitle layout and line segmentation. Two-line L1 subtitles appeared easier to process by viewers (d'Ydewalle and De Bruycker, 2007). Ill-segmented two-line subtitles, however, were fixated for slightly longer amounts of time than well-segmented ones, and correlated with slightly better overall comprehension of the audiovisual text (Perego et al., 2010). The trend relates ill-segmentation to depth of processing, and suggests another possible link with perceptual salience. In parallel to what has been claimed for subtitle translation, it can be hypothesized that high-quality subtitles do guarantee smoother reading, but may result in a shallower and less attentive encoding process. According to this interpretation, participants may have paid slightly more attention to ill-segmented subtitles, and this may actually have improved their capacity to encode information and grasp the gist of the part of the movie that was more difficult to follow.

On the whole, learning-oriented considerations and empirical findings seem to suggest that a stimulus to both faster and more attentive processing can be beneficial to L2 acquisition. The processes would aid learning based on opposite cognitive mechanisms, namely processing easification or the disruption of smooth processing through the enhancement of input components.

The two phenomena may prove to be most suitable for different categories of learners, for instance learners at different proficiency levels in the L2. Processing easification, as achieved through the addition of overtly cohesive subtitles, a low degree of linguistic variation from the ST, and a coherent line segmentation, might be advisable for beginning learners, who need to devote most of their cognitive resources to comprehension and are not yet able to operate elaborate mapping between ST and TT. Conversely, less smooth processing ensuing from a larger extent of divergence between ST and TT or ill-segmentation of subtitles could be of greater assistance to learners at more advanced proficiency levels, who would be more capable of noticing layout and translational "irregularities" thanks to their more holistic perception of the audiovisual text.

Future work that applies eye-movement methodology to the study of subtitled input consumption by language learners could prove helpful for tracing a more detailed picture of how subtitles are actually processed by this ever growing category of users as opposed to general audience. Such a line of research could shed light on which specific features of subtitled input, besides prolonged exposure to it, are likely to have a significant impact on the intake and acquisition of linguistic input – and thus define learner-specific usability features of subtitles.

References

Appiah, K. A. (2000), Thick Translation. In L. Venuti (ed.), *The Translation Studies Reader*. London: Routledge, 417–29.

Brondeel, H. (1994), Teaching Subtitling Routines. *Meta* 39(1), 26–33.

Caffrey, C. (2008a), Using Pupillometric, Fixation-Based and Subjective Measures to Measure the Processing Effort Experienced when Viewing Subtitled TV Anime with Pop-Up Gloss. In S. Göpferich, A. L. Jakobsen and I. M. Mees (eds), *Looking at Eyes. Eye-Tracking Studies of Reading and Translation Processing* [Special Issues]. *Copenhagen Studies in Language* 36, 125–44.

—— (2008b), Viewer Perception of Visual Nonverbal Cues in Subtitled TV Anime. *European Journal of English Studies* 12(2), 163–78.

Chaparro, B. S., A. D. Shaikh and J. R. Baker (2005), Reading Online Text with a Poor Layout: Is Performance Worse? *Usability News* 7. <http://psychology.wichita. edu/surl/usabilitynews/71/page_setting.asp> (accessed 14/10/2010)

Coltheart, M. (ed.) (1987), *Attention and Performance 2: The Psychology of Reading*. London: Lawrence Erlbaum.

Craig, J., and I. K. Scala (2006), *Designing with Type, the Essential Guide to Typography*. New York: Watson Guptil.

Danan, M. (2004), Captioning and Subtitling: Undervalued Language Learning Strategies. *Meta* 49(1), 67–77.

De Linde, Z., and N. Kay (1999), *The Semiotics of Subtitling*. Manchester: St Jerome.

Díaz-Cintas, J. (2003), *Teoría y prática de la subtitulación. Inglés-Español*. Barcelona: Ariel Cine.

—— (ed.) (2008), *The Didactics of Audiovisual Translation*. Amsterdam: John Benjamins.

Díaz-Cintas, J., and G. Anderman (2009), *Audiovisual Translation: Language Transfer on Screen*. Basingstoke: Palgrave Macmillan.

Díaz-Cintas J., and M. Fernández Cruz (2008), Using Subtitled Video Materials for Foreign Language Instruction. In J. Díaz-Cintas (ed.), *The Didactics of Audiovisual Translation*. Amsterdam: John Benjamins, 201–14.

Díaz-Cintas J., P. Orero and A. Remael (2007), *Media for All: Subtitling for the Deaf, Audio Description, and Sign Language*. Amsterdam: Rodopi.

d'Ydewalle, G., and W. De Bruycker (2007), Eye Movements of Children and Adults While Reading Television Subtitles. *European Psychologist* 12(3), 196–205.

d'Ydewalle, G., and I. Gielen (1992), Attention Allocation with Overlapping Sound, Image, and Text. In K. Rayner (ed.), *Eye Movements and Visual Cognition*. Berlin: Springer-Verlag, 415–27.

d'Ydewalle, G., C. Praet, K. Verfaillie and J. Van Rensbergen (1991), Watching Subtitled Television. Automatic Reading Behaviour. *Communication Research* 18(5), 650–66.

d'Ydewalle, G., J. Van Rensbergen and J. Pollet (1987), Reading a Message When the Same Message is Available Auditorily in Another Language: The Case of Subtitling. In J. K. O'Regan and A. Lévy-Schoen (eds), *Eye Movements: From Psychology to Cognition*. Amsterdam: North-Holland, 313–21.

d'Ydewalle, G., L. Warlop and J. Van Rensbergen (1989), Television and Attention: Differences Between Young and Older Adults in the Division of Attention Over Different Sources of TV Information. *Medienpsychologie: Zeitschrift für Individual- und Massenkommunikation* 1, 42–57.

Ghia, E. (2007), A Case Study on the Role of Interlingual Subtitles on the Acquisition of L2 Syntax – Initial Results. In A. Baicchi (ed.), *Voices on Translation. Linguistic, Multimedia, and Cognitive Perspectives* [Special Issue]. *RILA* 39, 167–77.

—— (forthcoming), The Impact of Translation Strategies on Subtitle Reading. In E. Perego and G. d'Ydewalle (eds), *Broadening the Horizons in AVT. Eye Tracking-Based Studies on the Perception and Accessibility of Subtitled Films*. Amsterdam: John Benjamins.

Göpferich, S., A. L. Jakobsen and I. M. Mees (eds) (2008), Looking at Eyes: Eye Tracking Studies of Reading and Translation Processing [Special Issue]. *Copenhagen Studies in Language* 36.

Grimes, T. (1991), Mild Auditory-Visual Dissonance in Television News May Exceed Viewer Attentional Capacity. *Human Communication Research* 18, 268–98.

Henderson, J. M., M. Singer and F. Ferreira (eds) (1995), *Reading and Language Processing*. Mahwah and Hove: Lawrence Erlbaum.

Ivarsson, J. (2009), Bibliography of Subtitling and Related Subjects. <http://www.transedit.se/Bibliography.htm> (accessed 24/11/2010)

——, and M. Carroll (1998) *Subtitling*. Simrishamn: TransEdit HB.

James, H., I. Roffe and D. Thorne (1996), Assessment and Skills in Screen Translation. In C. Dollerup and V. Appel (eds), *Teaching Translation and Interpreting 2. Insights, Aims, Visions*. Amsterdam: John Benjamins, 177–86.

Karamitroglou, F. (1998), A Proposed Set of Subtitling Standards in Europe. *Translation Journal* 2(2).

Kothari, B. (2000), Same Language Subtitling on Indian Television: Harnessing the Power of Popular Culture for Literacy. In K. Wilkins (ed.), *Redeveloping*

Communication for Social Change: Theory, Practice and Power. New York: Rowman and Littlefield, 135–46.

Krashen, S. D. (1985), *The Input Hypothesis.* London: Longman.

Kruger, J. L. (2008), Subtitler Training as Part of a General Training Programme in the Language Professions. In J. Díaz-Cintas (ed.), *The Didactics of Audiovisual Translation.* Amsterdam: John Benjamins, 71–87.

LaBerge, D., and S. J. Samuels (1974), Toward a Theory of Automatic Information Processing in Reading. *Cognitive Psychology* 6, 293–323.

Lang, A. (2000), The Limited Capacity Model of Mediated Message Processing. *Journal of Communication* 50, 46–70.

Markham, P., and L. Peter (2002), The Influence of English Language and Spanish Language Captions on Foreign Language Listening/Reading Comprehension. *Journal of Educational Technology Systems* 31(3), 331–41.

Moran, S. (2008, June), The Effect of Linguistic Variation on Subtitle Reception. Paper presented at the international conference *Audiovisual Translation: Multidisciplinary Approaches*, University of Montpellier 3, France.

Nobili, P. (1995), Cinema(to)grafo. L'uso didattico dei sottotitoli per l'apprendimento delle lingue straniere. *SILTA – Studi Italiani di Linguistica Teorica e Applicata* 1, 151–72.

Perego, E. (2008), What Would We Read Best? Hypotheses and Suggestions for the Location of Line Breaks in Film Subtitles. *The Sign Language Translator and Interpreter* 2(1), 35–63.

——, F. Del Missier, M. Porta and M. Mosconi (2010), The Cognitive Effectiveness of Subtitle Processing. *Media Psychology* 13(3), 243–72.

Perfetti, C. A. (1985), *Reading Ability.* New York: Oxford Press.

Rayner, K., and A. Pollatsek (1987), Eye Movements in Reading: A Tutorial Review. In M. Coltheart (ed.), *Attention and Performance 12: The Psychology of Reading.* London: Lawrence Erlbaum, 327–62.

——(1989), *The Psychology of Reading.* Englewood Cliffs, NJ: Prentice Hall.

Reichle, E. D., A. Pollatsek and K. Rayner (2007), Modeling the Effects of Lexical Ambiguity on Eye Movements during Reading. In R. P. G. van Gompel, M. H. Fischer, W. S. Murray and R. L. Hill (eds), *Eye Movements: A Window on Mind and Brain.* Oxford: Elsevier, 271–92.

Sanders, M. S., and E. J. McCormick (1993), *Human Factors in Engineering and Design.* Blacklick: McGraw-Hill.

Sharwood-Smith, M. (1993), Input Enhancement in Instructed SLA: Theoretical Bases. *Studies in Second Language Acquisition*, 15, 165–79.

Smith, F. (2004), *Understanding Reading.* Hillsdale, NJ: Lawrence Erlbaum.

Smith, S. (1998), The Language of Subtitling. In Y. Gambier (ed.), *Translating for the Media*. Turku: Painosalama Oy, 139–49.

Tanenhaus, M. K. (2007), Eye Movements and Spoken Language Processing. In R. P. G. van Gompel, M. H. Fischer, W. S. Murray and R. L. Hill (eds), *Eye Movements: A Window on Mind and Brain*. Oxford: Elsevier, 444–69.

Tveit, J. E. (2004), *Translating for Television. A Handbook in Screen Translation*. Bergen: J. K. Publishing.

Van de Poel, M., and G. d'Ydewalle (2001), Incidental Foreign-Language Acquisition by Children Watching Subtitled Television Programs. In Y. Gambier and H. Gottlieb (eds), *(Multi)Media Translation. Concepts, Practices, and Research*. Amsterdam: John Benjamins, 259–73.

Van Lommel, S., A. Laenen and G. d'Ydewalle (2006), Foreign-Grammar Acquisition While Watching Subtitled Television Programmes. *British Journal of Educational Psychology* 76, 243–58.

Verfaillie, K., and G. d'Ydewalle (1987), Modality Preference and Message Comprehension in Deaf Youngsters Watching TV. *Psychological Report* 70.

NOA TALAVÁN ZANÓN

A Quasi-experimental Research Project on Subtitling and Foreign Language Acquisition

1. Introduction

Learning foreign languages with the help of audiovisual materials (in the form of video) brings language to life, because audiovisual input is connected to a recreational part of everyday life. These resources drive students towards credible and realistic situations, which do not belong to conventional language teaching scenarios, limited in terms of time and space. In this context, the inclusion of subtitling can foster the intrinsic benefits of (semi-authentic) video, and provide a motivation boost when students realize that when they use subtitles, they can understand and retain the foreign language better.

Today, the new technological resources of the Western world, such as digital and satellite TV or DVD/Blu-ray, allow the audience to choose their language and subtitles for each and every film, TV series or documentary they want to watch. Likewise, the ever growing presence of computers in nearly every home makes the practice of subtitling (the addition of subtitles by students) increasingly feasible both inside and outside the classroom context. Therefore, failure to use such technology to improve foreign language learning (FLL) in general, and English in particular, can be considered as a waste of resources.

This article will describe a quasi-experimental research project that was carried out to assess the benefits of both the activity of subtitling – i.e. the creation of interlingual subtitles by students themselves – and the use of ready-made subtitles as a support in order to enhance listening comprehension (LC) of audiovisual content.

2. Listening comprehension

LC is a very relevant skill in FLL. According to Buck (2001), 45% of our communication time is devoted to listening. Besides, this receptive skill is very complex, given that different types of processes (neurological, linguistic, pragmatic and psycholinguistic) take place in the individual when he/she hears an oral text. Unfortunately, LC has been neglected in foreign language (FL) education for many years, precisely because of its intrinsic complexity that makes it a very difficult skill to teach. However, this situation has considerably improved in recent times thanks to the work of several authors (Brown, 1995; Buck, 2001; Rost, 2002), who have claimed its relevance, analysed its components thoroughly, and suggested diverse strategies for its proper acquisition. It should not be forgotten that this skill is one of the pillars of real life communication, as well as one of FLL aspects students usually find most difficult to develop.

Defining LC is not easy because it is an intangible mental process and that is why it is often explained by means of metaphors or analogies. Besides, it is a very subjective process, whereby a particular person builds the global meaning of an oral text, so that it is influenced by multiple factors relative to the person creating the message and the time when it is produced; it even depends on the type of text and on the situation where it is inserted. Rost (2002) says that there are as many definitions of LC as types of this skill and, in order to better understand it, this author provides four categories around which the possible definitions of LC can be grouped: receptive (the reception of individual words on the part of the hearer), constructive (the construction and representation of the message), negotiative (the negotiation of the meaning with the speaker and the answer provided), and transformative (the creation of meaning through participation, imagination and empathy).

This project centres on the second type: constructive LC. This skill is analysed unilaterally (with no speaker involved, since students try to understand audiovisual content), so that transformative and negotiative focus are absolutely out of the picture. As to receptive LC, the use of subtitles and subtitling requires understanding of global messages and not individual words and expressions; that is why, this type of LC is not included here either. Thus, a definition of this skill adapted to the goals of the present research project could be the following: "listening means reframing the speaker's message in a way that's relevant to you" (Rost, 2002: 2).

3. Theoretical basis

The didactic benefits of subtitling as an active task and subtitles as a support is backed up by three relevant theories that explain how the brain processes input, particularly in terms of multimedia input: (1) the Cognitive Theory of Multimedia Learning, (2) the Dual Coding Theory and (3) the Theory of Information Processing.

Firstly, the Cognitive Theory of Multimedia Learning (Mayer, 2003) explains how individuals possess a limited capacity to pay attention to input when it comes from one channel only (for example, oral). However, if a second channel is added (for example, visual), bringing about extra related information, this limited capacity of information processing is expanded. If a third channel is added to the picture (for example, textual), as happens when subtitling is involved, the possibilities of information processing are widened even more, and previous knowledge activation becomes easier (Wang and Chen, 2007). When the cognitive load is reduced thanks to the connections established among the different channels, and between the textual information and previous knowledge, LC is facilitated. According to Jones and Plass (2002: 557), in their study on the possible forms of support (written, visual, both etc.) from the perspective of the Cognitive Theory of Multimedia Learning:

> When students listened to an oral passage, they understood the narration better and learned more vocabulary when they selected from the pictorial and written annotations that were available for keywords in the narration than when they selected only one type of annotation or none.

Secondly, according to the Dual Coding Theory (Paivio, 1991), information is processed and saved by means of two different (though related)
memory systems: visual and verbal. That is the reason why, when verbal
information is accompanied by images, students are capable of building
referential connections between these two forms of mental representation
and so they can learn more efficiently. Information is thus better and faster
retained when it is coded in a dual mode, through both memory systems.
In this sense, subtitles as a support and subtitling as the active creation of
subtitles include an additional verbal mode, the written form, that links
the verbal (oral) and the visual ones, so as to facilitate LC and language
retention.

The last theory to be mentioned is Information Processing Theory,
according to which, memory possesses three storage structures: sensory
memory, short-term memory and long-term memory. The first stage of
information processing takes place in the sensory memory, where individuals receive the information through all the sensory receptors. Then, once
this type of information is recognized, it is stored only in a visual and/
or verbal mode, that is, through the two main types of sensory memory:
iconic (for visual information) and echoic (for verbal stimuli). This information moves from here to the short-term memory, and whatever is retained
throughout a long period of time ends up in the long-term memory. What
is relevant for this research is that the first two filters of information in this
process are precisely visual and verbal, and the three channels involved
(images, audio and text) when audiovisual material and subtitling are used
in FLL are precisely those two enhanced by a replication of one of them:
the written form connected to the oral text by means of translation (be it
interlingual or intralingual). Wang and Shen (2007: online) summarize
the relevance of this theory when subtitles (or captions) are involved in
the following chart:

Figure 3: FLL through video and subtitles

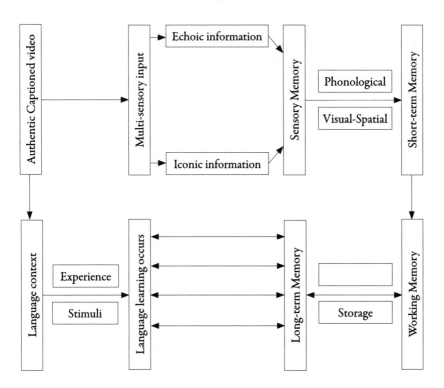

4. Previous research

Although there is not yet a thorough bibliography on the use of this tool in FLL, a series of interesting studies and proposals have appeared over the last decades. This review of previous research must be divided into two separate blocks, the use of ready-made subtitles as a support (where there is already an interesting bulk of research) and the more recent field of subtitling *per se*, which is, the addition of subtitles by students as an active task.

Subtitles as a support have been studied from different perspectives, depending on the main types employed: subtitles for the deaf and hard-of-hearing (SDH), bimodal and standard subtitles.

SDH are similar to bimodal subtitles (both the oral and the written text contain the FL), but they also contain paralinguistic information (sounds, for example) and they differentiate the voices of the various characters through colours or by means of their position on screen. In the United States they are known as closed captions and they have been very useful for the immigrant population in better understanding foreign television (Parks, 1994; Huang, 1999). As a matter of fact, the most relevant studies on the pedagogical use of SDH discuss the power of this type of support in enhancing second language learning, especially in the case of immigrants: Adler (1985), Parlato (1986), Huffman (1986), National Captioning Institute (1990), Smith (1990), Spanos (1990), Koskinen et al. (1991, 1993, 1996), Neuman and Koskinen (1992), and Gómez (2003).

Bimodal subtitles, on the other hand, contain the FL both in the audio and in the text. They have been used for years in FLL with very good results in terms of oral comprehension (Garza, 1991; Gant, 1998; Caimi, 2006; Talaván, 2010), oral production (Borrás and Lafayette, 1994; Araújo, 2008), reading comprehension (Bravo, 2008) and vocabulary learning (Vanderplank, 1988; Bird and Williams, 2002). However, it must be noted that when bimodal subtitles are used with total beginners, they can end up being too complex given that these students usually lack the necessary reading speed to follow them. Other authors who have studied the advantages of bimodal subtitles are: Blane (1996), Baltova (1999), Chung (1999), Markham (1999), Yoshino et al. (2000), Hervás (2001), and Mitterer and McQueen (2009).

Standard subtitles are the most commonly known subtitles and are most widely used in FLL; this is because they are easiest to follow, given that the audio is in the FL, but the text is in the viewer's mother tongue. Thus, it becomes very valuable for comprehension of the video input, as the student can establish connections between both linguistic systems, by means of translation and his previous knowledge of the target language. Standard subtitles help the student deal with authentic input from the very first day of the learning process, and increase confidence when dealing with similar types of authentic communicative exchanges in the FL. Standard subtitles have been found to be useful especially in terms of vocabulary development (Pavakanun and d'Ydewalle, 1992; Koolstra and Beentjes, 1999; Van de Poel and d'Ydewalle, 2001), and general linguistic skills for elementary levels (Araújo, 2008).

Last but not least, as far as subtitling as a task in FLL is concerned, previous research is rather scarce. Williams and Thorne (2000) found it useful to develop various skills, mainly LC, vocabulary, writing and cultural-historical knowledge. A European project has created a subtitling tool specially designed to use this task in FLL: *LvS* or *Learning via Subtitling* (Sokoli, 2006; Sokoli et al., this volume), a program being piloted at the moment all around Europe. Finally, other studies have been performed pertaining to the use of subtitling to improve translating skills (Neves, 2004; McLoughlin, 2009), although they are not discussed in this paper.

5. The project: Participants, resources, design and procedures

As stated in the introduction, this study attempts to analyse the influence of subtitling in enhancing LC skills in FLL students; subtitling in terms of both the use of subtitles as a support and the active task of subtitling. Thus, two main research hypotheses can be derived: students of English as a FL can considerably improve LC skills thanks to the practice of authentic video clip subtitling within a multimedia environment and following a task-based communicative approach (main hypothesis) and viewing subtitled video clips can considerably improve posterior comprehension of similar viewings, within a multimedia environment and following a task-based communicative approach (secondary hypothesis). To assess the validity of the previous hypotheses, a transversal quasi-experimental model, using both qualitative and quantitative techniques, was designed.

Before undertaking this project, two previous related research studies had been carried out so as to design the final model as reasonably and rigorously as possible. The first study analysed just the use of subtitles as a support for the development of oral skills (in terms of comprehension, production and interaction) from a qualitative point of view. Among the main conclusions, it was interesting to note students' positive reactions, the improvement of LC skills and the oral reproduction of communicative expressions related to the clips watched. The second preliminary study explored the possibility of carrying out a didactic strategy focused on the use of subtitles as a support and subtitling as a strategy to improve LC skills. The feasibility of such an approach (as far as time and resources were concerned) was qualitatively confirmed and students' reactions to the continuous use of such an activity seemed quite promising.

Hence, the realization of the pilot study of the final research was made possible thanks to the conclusions and experience obtained in the previous studies. Finally, the pilot study, which validated the initiation of the final research and revealed some shortcomings that led to a series of modifications in the final approach, was carried out.

To understand the final quasi-experimental study, a series of aspects must be described: participants, resources, the methodological construct, and procedures.

The participants were 50 adult subjects enrolled in the Official School of Languages in Spain (English as a FL level A2, studying B1). They were randomly divided in two groups, Experimental group and Control group (each one with a similar number of 25 subjects), and they received similar lessons focused on the use of bimodal subtitles as support (both groups were exposed to the second hypothesis), and subtitling as an active learning task (only group E undertook this activity). Given that selection was random, the population studied does not ensure complete statistical equivalence between groups C and E; this non-equivalence is rather common in quasi-experimental pedagogical studies. Nevertheless, an acceptable partial control is kept, considering that students attend the same course in the same language centre, have the same level of English, and live in the same town. In fact, the level of students, one of the most relevant factors in this type of pedagogical research, is sufficiently monitored because the school they attend is a national institution that controls the students' access to each and every course through standardized exams.

As far as resources are concerned, in this study they can be divided in two groups: computer related and questionnaires. As regards hardware, the research took place in a computer room and utilized a total number of 25 computers with Windows XP as the operating system. In terms of software, the main computer programs used were Subtitle Workshop, DVD Shrink, and Class Perfect. The first one was installed in all the computers so that group E could carry out the subtitling task. This particular subtitling program was chosen because it is freeware (students can continue to use it at home) and it has a very flexible, easy and attractive interface. The second program listed, DVD Shrink, was used by the researcher to edit the video clips used in the course of the lesson and it is also freeware. Finally, Class Perfect is a more complex program that was used by the teacher to monitor students' computers, by sending them the videos and particular instructions and by capturing each computer's screen when necessary.

As far as the questionnaire is concerned, a research tool very commonly used in social sciences, it was used in this study in order to perform a statistical definition of the population sample, as well as to reach qualitative conclusions as to general practices related to the tools and the tasks used. It was a self-completion questionnaire with a mixed design (most questions were closed but there was a final open item). While Robson (2002) recommends closed questions in self-completion questionnaires, Cohen et al. (2007: 330) claim that open questions can contain "the 'gems' of information that otherwise might not be caught in the questionnaire [and] can catch the authenticity, richness, depth of response, honesty and candour which [...] are the hallmarks of qualitative data".

In the field of research in LC, Buck (2001) recommends talking about the methodological construct, as the union of the text, the test and the theoretical approach.

The texts, in this case, were audiovisual in the form of two short video clips (two minutes approximately) related in content. Thus, these texts are semi-authentic, since they are originally created for native speakers and, even if they follow a script, they are supposed to exhibit natural (almost authentic) speech. They were taken from a popular sitcom and selected based on the following criteria: suitability for students' FLL level, previous knowledge about the sitcom unnecessary, independency of the communicative situation, interest and appropriateness of the topic, visual-oral correlation, and existence of humoristic elements.

LC tests consisted of a summary of the main ideas students could understand from each scene. Learners were asked to relate the story to a friend who missed that part of the series. Groups E and C viewed the scenes twice accompanied by bimodal subtitles while taking notes and after the second viewing they were told to write all the ideas they could remember from the clip in their mother tongue in the form of a summary. This is one of the most objective types of LC test according to Buck (2001) and Rost (2002), since no subjective questions are formulated in advance and students simply account for the communicative messages they have understood in their own language, so that there is no interference of other skills; LC solely. The assessment was prepared in terms of the total number of "idea units" (Buck, 2001: 9) students were able to understand. Each clip or text was analysed by several observers until a total amount of 15 idea units per video clip were used as the template for correction.

Regarding the theoretical approach, this project utilizes communicative task-based theories for its general framework. Since it focuses on LC in particular, the theoretical approach must be described in terms of the definition of LC chosen, the relationship between the participants, the situation, teacher and student roles and the assessment approach followed. The definition of LC chosen is constructive LC, as explained above; that is, the construction and representation of the message (idea units). The relationship between the speaker and the hearer is one way in this case, since there is no interaction, as happens in most LC tests; a positive aspect of assessing non-collaborative LC is that it minimizes the existence of other variables related to interaction skills. Regarding the communicative situations that appear in the clips, they are everyday situations that do not require the understanding of any specific socio-cultural elements and could take place in any country. In terms of roles, the teacher just monitored and guided the fluent progress of the tasks, helping to make comprehension meaningful, while the student was the one in control of the task, both deciding which elements to include in the LC tests (groups C and E), and subtitling the second clip (group E only). Last but not least, the assessment approach was both integrative and communicative, following Buck's (2001) classification. It is integrative because it includes the summary of ideas and some form of translation (since the summary is in the student's mother tongue); it is communicative also as it utilizes semi-authentic language and possesses a clear communicative goal: to relate the scene viewed to a friend when requested to do so.

Finally, the form of the lessons must be explained. Classes lasted 60 minutes. There was a preliminary warm-up (5 minutes) followed by viewing of the first clip with bimodal subtitles. Students watched the clip twice while taking notes (5') and they had 5 more minutes to write the summary. After this, group E undertook the task of subtitling (25'), into their mother tongue, the clip they had just summarized, individually on their computers with guidance and assistance from the teacher if required; at the end of this stage, one of the subtitled clips was chosen so that the whole group could see the final result of one random member of the class. Meanwhile, group C discussed the contents of the first clip (25'), its comprehension, and particularly difficult lexical items with the help of the teacher, and they watched the clip, now without subtitles, three more times interspersed with discussion. This parallel work was designed this way so that the amount of FL input and work was balanced between both groups, the only difference being the subtitling task performed by group E. Then, the two groups watched the second clip twice with bimodal subtitles (this clip was related in terms of characters and contexts to the first one) while they took notes for the subsequent summary (10'). Finally, a discussion similar (but shorter) to the one undertaken by group C with the previous clip was carried out by both groups, as a post-viewing activity to close the lesson (10'). The completion of questionnaires took place afterwards (5').

6. Results and discussion

A quasi-experimental research project presents a mixture of quantitative and qualitative methods. In this case, the quantitative stage contains the description of the participants sample, describes a series of correlation studies undertaken and analyses the results of the hypothesis test. The qualitative stage, on the other hand, is organized around the tools of data collection: observation and questionnaires.

Therefore, as part of the quantitative examination, the participants' sample is described from the point of view of the individuals, the use of AVT applications, and their reactions to the activity performed. The population sample is composed of adult students of English as a FL, with a medium-high socio-cultural level. They are all Spanish native speakers, most studying or who have studied another FL. Therefore, it is a homogeneous sample that, furthermore, is interested in the use of audiovisual materials; consequently the research results will have a sufficient level of generalization. Regarding the use of AVT applications, 74% of students claim that they use subtitles as a support at home (although not in class), especially bimodal ones; thus, they are already quite motivated in this regard. However, only a small group of students (20%) had practiced active subtitling previously, which means that this aspect of the study was new to most. In terms of participants' reactions to the activity, it can be noted that 86% of students consider it useful or very useful, 92% believe that this type of support enhances LC in a relevant way, while 86% believe that subtitling can also help to positively develop this skill.

Later, a series of correlation studies are considered so as to check the level of independence of the test results and the participants' sample. For this, some variables that describe the participants' sample were correlated with the results of the LC tests. Fortunately, there is no correlation in any of the cases analysed, so that it was inferred that both (the participants sample and the results) work independently; hence, it is assured that the results can be safely extrapolated.

The last part of the quantitative analysis is devoted to hypotheses testing; these tests are performed statistically using the LC test results of both groups (E and C). In test 1 (from clip 1) the average of results of both groups is 5.8, with a standard deviation of 2.48, which makes distribution quite irregular.

Hence, the results are relatively low, bearing in mind that the test was assessed from 1 to 15 idea units understood. Fortunately, test 2 (from clip 2) shows a clear improvement, with an average of 6.6 for the whole sample of participants and a standard deviation of 2.98; besides, the distribution is much closer to a normal one in statistical terms.

Although it is not a totally "normal distribution", it contains more intermediate results (in a 1–15 scale) than extreme ones. This preliminary characterization analysis of results of the whole sample leads to suspect that the use of subtitles as support in the first test is significant for the comprehension of the second one, a fact that would confirm the secondary hypothesis.

When this analysis is undertaken considering the answers of groups C and E independently, the results are more reveling. Group C average in test 2 is 5.9, with a standard deviation of 3.2.

Here, the distribution is not very close to normal, since the values are closer to extremes than to intermediate points; however, although there is not an obvious improvement from test 1, there are more intermediate results than in test 1, and some marks are evidently higher. Nevertheless, the real contrast is clearly seen in the results of group E in test 2, where the average of results is 7.3 (from 5.8 obtained by the whole sample in test 1), the standard deviation also diminishes to 2.6 and the distribution is much closer to "normal" than the ones commented before.

In this case, all marks (except the ones at both extremes) are covered by a certain number of subjects, specially the intermediate ones and some above the average. Consequently, there is a distinct improvement when compared with group C. With a higher average and a lower standard deviation, it can be tentatively concluded that there is an intrinsic relationship between subtitling as a task and LC improvement (which would confirm the main hypothesis), that leads the way for the hypothesis test.

The hypothesis test performed in this research project is a unilateral one, since it considers that participants can only improve in their results, that is, there is only one direction possible. The calculation criteria established for the statistical values is the difference of averages, that is, the hypothesis test is based on the comparison of averages obtained by the sample in the LC tests. From this basis, the behaviour of averages in the population as a whole can be inferred through the generalization of results. Since the population as a whole is impossible to grasp, a statistical inference about reality is made from a representative sample: the present adult FLL students.

In order to address this test, two hypotheses were established: null hypothesis (H_o) and alternative or research hypothesis (H_l). The former implies that subtitling has had no influence whatsoever; the latter, on the other hand, suggests that active subtitling is relevant. Then, a normal distribution is assumed as $N(o.1)$, and it must be noted that the confidence level (N_C) chosen is connected to the level of statistical significance (N_S) and with the critical value (z_C), in the terms presented in Table 20.

Table 20: Confidence level and critical value

Confidence level N_C	90%	95%	99%
Critical value z_C	1.28	1.645	2.33

Hence, the value of each test is obtained from the following formula, which will be known as "expression 1":

$$z = \frac{(\bar{x}_B - \bar{x}_A) - (\mu_B - \mu_A)}{\sqrt{\dfrac{\sigma_A^2}{N} + \dfrac{\sigma_B^2}{N}}}$$

In the calculation, $\bar{x}_A$ and $\bar{x}_B$ are the averages of both groups, while μ_A and μ_B are the mathematical expectations as regards the population as a whole. The hypothesis test is performed in the following way: the null hypothesis (nothing changes) is admitted as true, that is, mathematical expectations are assumed to be equal: $\mu_A - \mu_B = o$. Thus, the former "expression 1" turns into the following formula, which will be named "expression 2":

$$z = \frac{(\bar{x}_B - \bar{x}_A)}{\sqrt{\dfrac{\sigma_A^2}{N} + \dfrac{\sigma_B^2}{N}}}$$

The value obtained for z is compared with the critical value z_C, and it can be observed if it is in or out of range, that is, if it is situated between o and z_C. If this is the case, the null hypothesis is true; if not, false. If the null hypothesis is false, the alternative hypothesis would be confirmed, proving that changes take place. "Expression 2" is used, thus, to assess the realization of both hypotheses. In the first place, to verify the influence of the textual support of subtitles (secondary hypothesis), the results of tests 1 and 2 are compared taking into account the whole sample of participants (see Table 21).

Table 21

	Test 1	Test 2
$\bar{x}$	5.8	6.6
σ	2.5	3

Using "expression 2", z equals 1.449, and this, according to the confidence level and critical value references described above, provides a confidence level (N_C) of 90% and a critical value (z_C) of 1.28. Therefore, the null hypothesis is rejected, confirming the alternative one: viewing subtitled video clips can considerably improve posterior comprehension of similar viewings; accordingly, the secondary hypothesis proves to be true with a 90% confidence level.

After that, "expression 2" is used to examine the influence of subtitling as a task in the enhancement of LC. This verification would validate the main hypothesis of this research. To this end, the results of group C in test 2 (no subtitling performed previously) are compared with those obtained by group E in this test (after practicing subtitling as a task).

Table 22

	Group C	Group E
$\bar{x}$	5.9	7.3
σ	3.2	2.6

Using, again, "expression 2" as a reference, it is obtained that the value z equals 1.698, which corresponds to a confidence level (N_C) of 95%, since the critical value (z_C) is 1.645 (following the reference levels above). Ergo, the null hypothesis is rejected once more, confirming the alternative one: students of English as a FL can considerably improve LC skills thanks to the practice of authentic video clip subtitling. In other words, the main hypothesis is ratified, given that there is an obvious influence of subtitling in LC improvement, with a 95% level of confidence.

Thanks to the hypothesis test and the preliminary analysis, the main research hypotheses are validated, in other words, the value of subtitles as support for comprehension and the value of subtitling as an active and dynamic strategy to improve LC are confirmed.

Now, the qualitative examination is organized around the instruments of data collection: observation, questionnaires and LC tests, as it was noted above.

The analysis regarding observation considers the notes taken by the researcher and the questionnaire results and observations, and compares them with the quantitative results above; this way, triangulation of results is achieved, providing a greater level of reliability to the conclusions derived. The study of observation concludes, basically, that there is a high degree of reliability in the selected research method and the observed data, that most participants show a relevant interest in the performance of similar activities, and that there is enough evidence to obtain analogous conclusions in a similar research, set about in a longitudinal mode.

The study of the data collected from the questionnaire and the LC tests is also combined with observation, so as to check the previous triangulation and to provide a higher degree of reliability for the experiment. After this analysis is performed, a series of tendencies in FL education are derived: participants capable of speaking other languages find it easier to improve LC skills; audiovisual materials and subtitles are very rarely used in the classroom; learners used to working with subtitles possess better LC skills than those who do not use this resource; A2 level students possess a relatively accurate appreciation of their own LC level; previous knowledge related to the video clips used enhances comprehension of the content; note-taking, as a learning strategy, can be useful in the development of

LC; the use of these resources related to audiovisual materials, ICT and subtitling encourages students to make wider use of this type of support. The mixture of quantitative and qualitative techniques and the use of triangulation render this study robust in terms of its reliability and the potential generalization of results. The following pedagogical implications can be derived from the data gathered and analysed: the researched strategy can foster the acquisition of a series of "can dos" related to audiovisual comprehension, it can encourage autonomous learning both inside and outside the classroom, it may promote the enhancement of other related language skills (specially reading comprehension and writing production), it strengthens the role of mediation in FL education, and it ratifies the relevance of note-taking and summary as learning strategies for LC.

All in all, the pedagogical use of authentic video and AVT applications related to subtitling motivates students to make more frequent individual use of these resources (related to ICT) that will help them to achieve progressive improvement of LC skills. More importantly, the suggested strategy (based on the use of subtitles and subtitling), that is set in a communicative task-based learning context, combines a series of qualities that motivate, foster, and facilitate LC acquisition: it is recreational, familiar and dynamic, utilizes multiple codes, and makes the achievement of various linguistic skills possible, both individually and collaboratively.

Nowadays, the consolidation of English as *lingua franca* requires new tools and teaching strategies that can cope with an increasingly growing market. In this sense, given that the goal of language teaching should be, as a general rule, to lead students to efficient communication (where one of the main aspects is LC), this quasi-experiment has studied how this can be achieved adopting AVT applications based on the use of subtitles as support and on the addition of subtitles by the students themselves. Ultimately, it is hoped that these resources will be integrated into the educational curricula and that publishing houses will encourage the development of related materials in FL education.

Although, as in any research study, there are a series of limitations related to the number of participants and observants or the temporal length of the study, such drawbacks can be resolved in future research, since there is no doubt that future studies will require clarifications in terms of form, choice of instruments and methodology, as well as assessment. Considering that there is no "miraculous", definite or global answer to FL pedagogy, a constant search for possible specific solutions will always be needed so as to cope with the immense diversity of learner profiles, requirements and circumstances. Obviously, undertaking research studies similar to this one is no easy task, be it in material, economic or technical terms. Yet all these efforts are essential to advance knowledge and widen research studies like the one presented here, as it represents a step forward in the discipline and deserves to be expanded in order to respond to the new questions raised by the answers provided.

References

Adler, R. (1985), Using Closed-Captioned Television in the Classroom. *New Directions in Reading: Research and Practice* 1, 11–18.

Araújo, V. (2008), The Educational Use of Subtitled Films in EFL Teaching. In J. Díaz-Cintas (ed.), *The Didactics of Audiovisual Translation*. Amsterdam: John Benjamins, 227–38

Baltova, I. (1999), Multisensory Language Teaching in a Multidimensional Curriculum: The Use of Authentic Bimodal Video in Core French. *Canadian Modern Language Review/La Revue Canadienne des Langues Vivante* 56(1), 31–48.

Bird, S., and J. Williams (2002), The Effect of Bimodal Input on Implicit and Explicit Memory: An Investigation into the Benefits of Within-Language Subtitling. *Applied Psycholinguistic* 23(04), 509–33.

Blane, S. (1996), Interlingual Subtitling in the Languages Degree. In P. Sewell and I. Higgins (eds), *Teaching Translation in Universities: Present and Future Perspectives*. London: Association for Foreign Language Studies and Centre for International Language Teaching Research, 183–207.

Borrás, I., and R. Lafayette (1994), Effects of Multimedia Courseware Subtitling on the Speaking Performance of College Students of French. *The Modern Language Journal* 78(1), 61–75.

Bravo, M. C. (2008), *Putting the Reader in the Picture. Screen Translation and Foreign-Language Learning*. Tarragona: Universitat Rovira I Virgili. Doctoral Thesis.

Brown, G. (1995), *Speakers, Listeners and Communication*. Cambridge: Cambridge University Press.

Buck, G. (2001), *Assessing Listening*, Cambridge: Cambridge University Press.

Caimi, A. (2006), Audiovisual Translation and Language Learning: The Promotion of Intralingual Subtitles. *The Journal of Specialised Translation* 6, 85–98.

Chung, J. (1999), The Effects of Using Video Texts Supported with Advance Organizers and Captions on Chinese College Students. *Foreign Language Annals* 32(3), 295–308.

Cohen, L., L. Manion and K. Morrison (2007), *Research Methods in Education*. London: Routledge.

Davis, R. (1998), Captioned Video: Making it Work for You. *The Internet TESL Journal* 4(3). <http://iteslj.org/Techniques/Davis-CaptionedVideo/> (accessed 14/05/2010).

De Bot, K., J. Jagt, H. Janssen, E. Kessels and E. Schils (1986), Foreign Television and Language Maintenance. *Second Language Research* 2(1), 72–82.

Gant, H. (1998), The Effects of Keyword Captions to Authentic French Video on Learner Comprehension. *CALICO Journal* 15(1–3), 89–109.

Garza, T. (1991), Evaluating the Use of Captioned Video Materials in Advanced Foreign Language Learning. *Foreign Language Annals* 24(3), 239–58.

Gómez, M. (2003), Un modelo de aprendizaje: La televisión por satélite para la elaboración de planes de clases en la enseñanza del inglés. *Anales de la Universidad Metropolitana* 3(2), 159–69.

Hervás, M. (2001), Subtitulado intralingüístico con fines didácticos. In L. Lorenzo and A. M. Pereira (eds), *El subtitulado: (inglés/español/gallego)*. Vigo: Servicio de publicaciones Universidad de Vigo, 147–68.

Huang, H. C. (1999), The Effects of Closed-Captioned Television on the Listening Comprehension of Intermediate English as a Second Language (ESL) Students. *Journal of Educational Technology System*, 28(1), 75–96.

Huffman, D. (1986), Soap Operas and Captioning in the EFL Class. Proceedings of the *International Conference on Language Teaching and Learning of the Japanese Association of Language Teachers*. Hamamatsu, Japan: Seirei Gakuen.

Jones, C., and J. L. Plass (2002), Supporting Listening Comprehension and Vocabulary Acquisition in French with Multimedia Annotations. *The Modern Language Journal* 86, 546–61.

Kumaravadivelu, B. (2005), *Understanding Language Teaching: From Method to Post-Method*. New York: Routledge.

Koolstra, C., and J. Beentjes (1999), Children's Vocabulary Acquisition in a Foreign Language through Watching Subtitled Television Programs at Home. *Educational Technology Research and Development* 47, 51–60.

Koskinen, P., J. Knable, P. Markham, C. Jensema and K. Kane (1996), Captioned Television and the Vocabulary Acquisition of Adult Second Language Correctional Facility Residents. *Journal of Educational Technology Systems* 24, 359–73.

Koskinen, P., R. Wilson, L. Gambrell and C. Jensema (1991), Captioned Video Technology and Television-Based Reading Instruction. In State of Maryland International Reading Association (ed.), *Literacy: Issues and Practice. Yearbook.* Maryland, MA: Bethesda, 39–47.

Koskinen, P., R. Wilson, L. Gambrell and S. Neuman (1993), Captioned Video and Vocabulary Learning: An Innovative Practice in Literacy Instruction. *The Reading Teacher* 47, 36–43.

Mayer, R. E. (2003), *Learning and Instruction.* New Jersey: Merrill/Prentice Hall.

McLoughlin, L. (2009), Subtitles in Translators' Training: A Model of Analysis. *Romance Studies* 27(3), 174–85.

Mitterer, H., and J. M. McQueen (2009), Foreign Subtitles Help but Native-Subtitles Harm Foreign Speech Perception. *PLoS One* 4(11). <http://www.ncbi.nlm.nih.gov/pmc/articles/PMC2775720/> (accessed 20/06/2010)

National Captioning Institute (1990), *Using Captioned Television to Improve the Reading Proficiency of Language Minority Students.* Falls Church, VA: National Captioning Institute.

Neuman, S., and P. Koskinen (1992), Captioned Television as Comprehensible Input: Effects of Incidental Word Learning from Context for Language Minority Students. *Reading Research Quarterly* 27, 94–106.

Neves, J. (2004), Language Awareness through Training in Subtitling. In P. Orero (ed.), *Topics in Audiovisual Translation.* Amsterdam: John Benjamins, 127–40.

Paivio, A. (1991), Dual Coding Theory: Retrospect and Current Status. *Canadian Journal of Psychology* 45, 255–87.

Parks, C. (1994), Closed Captioned TV: A Resource for ESL Literacy Education. *ERIC Digest*, ED 372 662. <http://www.ericdigests.org/1995-1/tv.htm> (accessed 26/11/2009).

Parlato, S. (1986), *Watch your Language: Captioned Media for Literacy.* Silver Spring, MD: T. J. Publishers.

Robson, C. (2002), *Real World Research: A Resource for Social Scientists and Practitioner-Researchers.* Oxford: Blackwell.

Rost, M. (2002), *Teaching and Researching Listening.* London: Longman.

Ryan, S. (1998), Using Films to Develop Learner Motivation. *The Internet TESL Journal* 4(11). <http://iteslj.org/Articles/Ryan-Films.html> (accessed 04/04/2010).

Smith, J. (1990), Closed-Caption Television and Adult Students of English as a Second Language. *ERIC Digest*, ED339 250.

Sokoli, S. (2006), Learning via Subtitling (LvS): A Tool for the Creation of Foreign Language Learning Activities Based on Film Subtitling. Proceedings *MuTra 2006 –Multidimensional Translation: Audiovisual Translation Scenarios.* Copenhagen: Copenhagen University, 66–73. <http://www.euroconferences.info/proceedings/2006_Proceedings/2006_Sokoli_Stravoula.pdf> (accessed 13/06/2010).

Spanos, G., and J. Smith (1990), Closed Captioned Television for Adult LEP Literacy Learners. *ERIC Digest*, ED 321 623. <http://www.ericdigests.org/pre-9216/closed.htm> (accessed 08/05/2010).

Talaván, N. (2010) Subtitling as a Task and Subtitles as Support: Pedagogical Applications. In J. Díaz-Cintas, A. Matamala and J. Neves (eds), *New Insights into Audiovisual Translation and Media Accessibility.* Amsterdam: Rodopi, 285–99.

Van de Poel, M., and G. d'Ydewalle (2001), Incidental Foreign-Language Acquisition by Children Watching Subtitled Television Programs. In Y. Gambier and H. Gottlieb (eds), *(Multi)Media Translation: Concepts, Practices and Research.* Amsterdam: John Benjamins, 259–74.

Wang, Y., and C. Shen (2007), Tentative Model of Integrating Authentic Captioned Video to Facilitate ESL Learning. *Sino-US English Teaching* 4(9). <http://www.linguist.org.cn/doc/su200709/su20070901.pdf> (accessed 01/05/2010).

Williams, H., and D. Thorne (2000), The Value of Teletext Subtitling as a Medium for Language Learning. *System* 28(2), 217–28.

Yoshino, S., K. Kano and K. Akahori (2000), The Effects of English and Japanese Captions on the Listening Comprehension of Japanese EFL Students. *Language Laboratory* 37, 111–30.

STAVROULA SOKOLI, PATRICK ZABALBEASCOA &
MARIA FOUNTANA

Subtitling Activities for Foreign Language Learning: What Learners and Teachers Think

1. Background

It is becoming increasingly evident to foreign language (FL) teachers and researchers that there is no single guaranteed teaching method and that a variety of materials, activities and technical resources may be used effectively in the classroom. The approach discussed in this paper concerns a combined use of videos, subtitles and Information and Communication Technologies (ICTs).

The advantages of video have been fully debated by teachers and researchers (Allan, 1985; Ciccone, 1995; King, 2002; Stempleski and Tomalin, 1990; Tschirner, 2001). Video offers variety, contextualizes linguistic items and provides exposure to cultural and nonverbal elements. As a means of communication, the audiovisual mode is closer to natural ideal communication than the written (printed or manuscript) or oral (radio, audio-cassette) modes (Zabalbeascoa, 2010). It can be argued that audio-only listening comprehension exercises have been devised due to technical constraints or lack of equipment (a VCR, when available was much more expensive than a tape-recorder in the 1980s). The recent availability of videos in DVD format, online libraries and video communities has led to an increasing use of this kind of material in FL classes. Alongside with the advantages of video, many issues have been raised about selection criteria for materials, degree of difficulty and learners' motivation, the principal question being: how to exploit videos for maximum efficiency? Watching a film and then answering questions about it is clearly using this resource optimally. A range of viewing activities have been suggested, such as silent viewing, freeze frame, role play, and prediction (Tomalin, 1990: 10–29). Subtitled videos have been regarded as particularly beneficial due to the function of subtitles as a bridge between reading and listening skills (Borrás and Lafayette, 1994). Numerous studies proving their usefulness have been conducted since the 1980s, an extensive account of which has been given by Gambier (2007). Depending on their relationship with the dialogue, subtitles can be standard, or interlingual, L2→L1; same-language or intralingual or bimodal (because of the combination of speaking and writing on the screen) L2→L2; and reversed (with regard to standard) L1→L2.[1] Standard subtitles are thought to help language learning without any conscious or systematic effort, especially in countries where subtitled television and cinema are widespread. In these so-called subtitling countries there is a popular belief that people acquire some knowledge of foreign languages incidentally, by watching television.[2] Finally, reversed subtitles have been proven to improve lexical skills, especially at beginner level (Danan, 1992).

The idea of asking language learners to add or modify subtitles on a video emerged with the view to enlarge the range of exploitable activities. The practice of subtitling implies involving the learners in a simulated real-world task whose outcome, unlike watching subtitles or using viewing techniques, is a tangible, shareable product: the subtitled video. The literature revealed that subtitling has been thought to improve translation learners' linguistic skills. This conclusion has been reached incidentally, as a side benefit of attending courses designed for future professionals (Klerkx, 1998; Williams and Thorne, 2000; Neves, 2004) using professional subtitling software (ScanTitling, the S4C subtitling suite, Screen-Win2020).

Subtitling for language learning is also closely related to the field of ICT in education. According to an analysis of the British Educational

---

1   L1→L1 subtitles are not discussed here because of their limited application in foreign language learning and teaching.

2   The EU funded project *Subtitles and Language Learning* (Life Long Learning Programme 2009–2012) led by the University of Turku aims to find further evidence.

Communications and Technology Agency (Becta),[3] ICT can contribute to foreign language skills acquisition and have positive effects both for pupils and teachers. More specifically, ICT contributes to the key FL skills of listening, speaking, reading and writing in a variety of ways, including access to a vast range of information and learning opportunities; personalized work rate as digital resources can be slowed and replayed repeatedly depending on individual needs; increased personal interest in FL by watching films in DVD format with subtitles and multiple audio tracks in different languages.

The desire to study the possibilities and limitations of subtitling in FLL engendered the Learning via Subtitling (LeViS) project and the development of the LvS software tool,[4] a subtitling simulator specifically designed for language learners' needs. LeViS was funded with support from the European Commission (Programme Socrates/Lingua II) from 2006 to 2008. Hellenic Open University coordinated the partnership which was formed by the Research Academic Computer Technology Institute (Greece), Transilvania University of Brasov (Rumania), University of the Algarve (Portugal), Roehampton University (UK), University of Pecs (Hungary) and Universidad Autónoma de Barcelona (Spain).

2. The LeViS project, software and activities

The main aim of the project Learning via Subtitling (<http://levis.cti.gr>) is to develop educational material and tools for active foreign language learning based on video subtitling. The project aims to cover the need for

---

3   Becta (<http://www.becta.org.uk>; accessed 16/06/2010) is the UK government-led agency for ICT in education and supports national organizations, schools and colleges in the use and development of ICT in education to raise standards, widen access, improve skills and encourage effective management.

4   The acronym LeViS is used to refer to the project and the approach. LvS refers to the software tool developed within the project framework.

active learning through task-based activities; cultural elements become authentic and motivating, and learners are exposed to highly contextualized language input.

The LeViS project included the following objectives:

- Design useful and attractive software for learners of some European languages which may not have received sufficient attention in FL learning and teaching.
- Propose lesson plans that would couch the software in a meaningful and carefully planned FLL environment.
- Test the software on actual students of the languages involved to draw conclusions both for improving methodological proposals and the software itself.
- Cross data from experiences and tests carried out in different countries, with different languages, learning styles, and student and teacher profiles, to draw conclusions regarding the applicability of translation exercises and activities in FLL.

This involved additional tasks that might also be considered as objectives:

- Design lesson plans that could fit in with recent trends and patterns in FL teaching and learning, and accommodate the centrepiece of the project, the LvS software for developing subtitling activities for FL students.
- Design questionnaires that would serve as an evaluation tool for measuring the success of the software and the outcome of the lesson plans.

A theoretical framework was established to serve as a basis for the software design and the development of materials. According to this framework, the LeViS approach is not a learning method designed to substitute current teaching practices, but rather an additional activity to enhance, or at least complement, them. The tool and learning activities are intended to be used at key points of a learning course and not necessarily on a regular basis. LeViS was based on the following hypotheses:

- Video, subtitling and ICT are useful in FLL.
- Learners using subtitling activities will be motivated by the process and the tangible result of their task.
- Motivation promotes learning and LeViS has an important motivational ingredient.

A subtitling simulator (LvS) has been designed for educational purposes in FLL. Through this tool and associated activities, the learner is asked to add subtitles to a film to engage in active listening and writing tasks.

Teachers can use the authoring mode of this software tool to create activities and learners can employ it to carry out tasks ranging from gap-filling to sorting shuffled subtitles, and from transcribing the utterances to translating them and even reauthoring.

The LvS main screen (Figure 4) is divided into four basic areas:

- The Video Player area allows viewing, rewinding and forwarding the video, with or without subtitles.
- The Document Viewer area is used for viewing the instructions and other files necessary for the activity (information about the clips, scripts, exercises etc.)
- The Subtitle Editor area is for editing and managing subtitles. Each subtitle line is divided into four columns: start and end time (the temporal points in the clip when the subtitle text appears on screen and disappears), duration, and subtitle text. Two more columns can be used for teacher and learner comments. The teacher can mark the subtitle line with icons for "well done", "warning", etc. which can be clicked on and take a student to the Notes Area.
- The Notes Area allows learners and teachers to exchange feedback. It is divided into general notes and comments per subtitle.

Figure 4: LvS screenshot

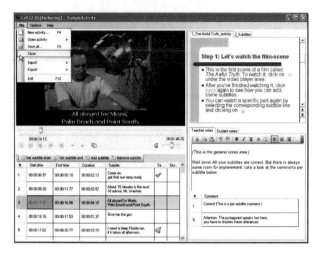

The flexibility in the use of LvS is evidenced in that it can be utilized in any real or virtual classroom and within any curriculum, as it does not imply any change in the methodology used. LvS is suitable for use in autonomous learning environments, since the interface includes a document viewer area, where all the necessary steps for self-study can be provided by the author of the activity. It can also be used in distance learning, as it includes feedback tools in the form of a general notes area and a comment per subtitle tool. Additionally, it may be employed for any number of learners, with unlimited choice of video content (film scenes, educational material), for any suitable duration of video segment, student level (beginners, intermediate, advanced), age and interests.

The approach adopted for LeViS activities was a combination of the instructional sequences known as the pre-, while-, post- procedure, and the TBL, or Task-Based Learning sequence. The first sequence aims at raising learners' awareness of and interest in a particular subject (pre-stage), undertaking a series of activities that involve these skills (while-stage) and evaluating and discussing these activities with reference to other skills (post-stage). The TBL sequence works on the assumption that focusing on language structure is not enough and that naturalistic exposure to and use of the language has to be prioritized.

A LeViS activity involves subtitle editing, but is otherwise similar to any other language learning activity. The term subtitling is used in an unusually broad sense here and does not necessarily involve all the steps in professional subtitling, such as spotting. It may also refer to adding captions to silent videos with no dialogue associated to the captions.

Depending on level and objectives, it may involve a variety of tasks. Beginners may be asked to put scrambled subtitles in the correct order, or in their right place. Intermediate learners may complete the blanks of existing subtitles, or use subtitles to describe the action and characters appearing in a video, for example. Activities for advanced learners may involve creating subtitles in L2 for dialogues in L1 or in L2. Technical constraints of subtitling, which require a maximum number of characters, help learners develop skills such as paraphrasing, abridging, finding synonyms, and choosing which linguistic elements to omit (Sokoli, 2006). In addition, if the activity demands meeting professional standards, learners must focus on syntactic and semantic structures in order to provide appropriate subtitle line division.

By introducing subtitling as an activity, the emphasis is not on the selection of the video but on what learners are asked to do with it. There may even be a video with no dialogue, as was the case with a home-made video used at Roehampton University. In addition, the choice of material is wider than in the past and not limited to film scenes extracted from a DVD. Apart from YouTube with its wide variety of channels, including the BBC and the Sundance channel, there are video resources such as the Internet Archive, Open Culture, EduTubePlus and Canal Educatif.

An example of an activity will be described here to illustrate the use of LeViS. The activity titled "The Awful Truth" aims at practicing listening skills and using the software itself. This lesson is planned for adults who learn English at beginner level (A2) with some basic computer skills or interest in using a computer. It is part of a course taking place in Greece, where subtitling is one of the most widely used modes of AVT. This means that learners are familiar with subtitles and they are in contact with English through watching subtitled AV programmes. The specific context of language learning justifies the use of subtitling in such an early stage of learning.

The warm-up activity (pre-stage), lasting 10–15 minutes, involves listening to the scene's dialogue without the image. Learners write down any words they recognize while listening. The teacher writes all the words on the board and explains that they will find out which of these words were actually heard in the next step of the activity.

The materials of the activity (while-stage) are:

- The instructions file, a PowerPoint presentation, which can be accessed through the Document Viewer area; it contains guidelines for the exercise and technical instructions on how the learners can copy and paste text.
- The video-clip, lasting 1 minute and 47 seconds, is the first scene from Leo McCarey's 1937 film The Awful Truth, starring Cary Grant and Irene Dunne. Its fast dialogue is difficult to understand for learners of this level but this scene contains phrases (greetings) they have already learned.
- A text file, containing the transcription of the dialogue in the form of mixed-up lines.

The learners watch the clip as many times as they like and read the transcription in the document viewer area of the software interface. They copy each line and paste it in the corresponding subtitle line in the subtitle area. This can be done either individually or in pairs. Eventually, the teacher provides the correct subtitle file and the learners compare it to their efforts.

It can be followed by a post-stage activity aimed at practising oral skills, where learners choose one of the characters, learn lines from the part of the dialogue and act it out in pairs.

The opportunities for using authentic listening material are limited at this level. However, it is made possible because of the nature of the activity which is simple and undemanding. Incidental learning is also expected to take place, since the learners have to listen to the video clip more than once (without being explicitly asked to) in order to carry out the task.

3. LeViS evaluation: Aim and methods

The aim of this evaluation is to investigate specific issues regarding the following areas:

- The LvS software focusing on usability and compliance with FLL approach.
- The educational activities, pertaining to the extent of use of activities, various ways of using activities, educational results (e.g. objectives met) and compliance with FLL approach.
- The language learning approach, specifically its validity (e.g. integrity with various curricula and classroom reality), utility (e.g. ease of use), added value (e.g. improves the quality of learning taking place), accuracy and reliability (with regard to the software on which it is based), documentation (teacher guidelines, student instructions, etc.)

The evaluation is based on the following general questions:

- Is the LvS software appropriate for language learning and teaching and under which circumstances?
- Are the language learning activities developed within the project appropriate for use in FLL curricula and according to which criteria?
- Are there any suggestions for project development and continuation?

To answer these general questions, evaluation was based on expert opinion, review of project outputs, but also on specific questions addressed to learners and teachers involved in the implementation phase of the project. The specific questions regarding teachers are summarized in the following list:

Background questions

- What is the teachers' perception of translation as a "tool" for FL teaching?
- What is the teachers' perception of using computer activities in FL teaching?

Evaluation questions

- What was the teachers' experience of using the LvS software and the activities?
- Were their teaching objectives met and if so, how (well)?
- How was the perception of success influenced by the way the activity was implemented and the level of teacher involvement in the development phase?

The questions concerning the learners are included in the following list:

Background question

- What was the learners' level of familiarity with FLL and computer activities in FLL?

Evaluation questions

- To what extent were learners involved in LeViS activities?
- What was learners' perception of the software and the activities?

The methods used for data collection included: (a) a combination of experimental and inquiry methods in order to evaluate the usability of the software; (b) questionnaires aimed at learners who used the software and the activities, and teachers (including activity authors and project members).

The usability evaluation took place at the Software Quality Assessment laboratory of the Hellenic Open University (Kostaras et al., 2010). The software was tested taking into consideration criteria such as functionality, interoperability, ease of use, accuracy and reliability, documentation available and compliance with the FLL approach. Most of the usability faults found were corrected in the final version of the software.

The present study focuses on the users' feedback, obtained exclusively through detailed analysis of their responses to the questionnaires, which were designed specifically for and within this project. Two different questionnaires were designed, one for learners and one for their teachers. The questions came with instructions for the informants (such as "tick-off the option that best describes what you think", "choose from 1 to 5"). Examples were offered where possible to clarify the questions. The questionnaires were translated and presented in the informants' native language.

Some of the questions were given with prompted answers, forming part of a numerical evaluation scale from 1 to 5. Verbal labels were given to explain the value or meaning of each number (1, 2, 3, 4 and 5) on the scale. The result was a mix of the "marking" number system, where the lower numbers, 1 and 2, were always negative (e.g. no, none, never, dislike, unhappy), 4–5 were positive (always, very much, very good), and 3 was meant as middle-of-the-road. The verbal labels were devised to help informants to score more unambiguously by marking and qualifying with words like "quite satisfied" or "very useful". Below, words that were prompted are signalled with an asterisk, and their numerical value is provided in brackets. For example, somewhat* (3/5) was for scoring three on a five-point scale, where value 3 was prompted by the word somewhat. A seven-point scale was used for only two questions.

4. Participants' profile and learning context

Teacher and Learner questionnaires were collected from the six countries where the project was implemented, involving 104 learners and 12 teachers. All learners were university students except the vocational school students in Romania. In total, 10 LeViS activities were taught in FL teaching classrooms for 8 languages and 15 sessions (see Table 23).

Table 23: Origin of evaluation data

Countries involved	6
Languages taught	8
LeViS Activities used	10
Classroom sessions	15
Learner questionnaires collected	104
Teacher questionnaires collected	12

Table 24 shows the breakdown of the project implementation and data collection.

Table 24: Breakdown of evaluation questionnaires collected

Participant country	Language taught	Learner questionnaires	Teacher questionnaires
Hungary	Hungarian	38	3
Romania	Romanian	10	1
UK	Spanish	3	1
Portugal	English	10	1
Greece	Greek	8	3
Spain	Portuguese	7	1
Spain	Italian	14	1
Spain	Chinese	14	1

Details of participants' profiles and the learning context are presented per country.

4.1. Hungary

The learners who filled in the questionnaires were second-year medical students (ages 20–22) of both genders and non-Hungarian origin. They were foreign learners studying at the Faculty of Medicine of Pecs University from countries like Norway, Sweden, Germany and Canada. They were studying Hungarian for medical purposes. Specifically, their working languages were English or German and they attended a Hungarian language learning course to enable them to communicate with Hungarian patients. When they answered the questionnaires they were in the 4th semester of the course (A2 level of competence).

All learners were very experienced in FLL since they all spoke four or five languages (including their mother tongue) on average. They were also very familiar with computer use for learning purposes (45% daily use), chatting (42% daily use) but also for shopping, reading news, watching films and playing games. However, they had no experience whatsoever of computer activities during their language learning classes and they were interested in trying more computer interaction in their FL classes. Most learners answered they had some experience with translation before doing any LeViS activity and almost all of them seemed to like translation as an activity. The same did not apply, though, to student experience in using video or multimedia as language learners.

The three tutors filling the questionnaires were all teachers of foreign languages (either English or German) at the Faculty of Medicine. In this particular context they taught Medical Hungarian as a foreign language to the informant learners. They all had some experience in translating (e.g. official translation of clinical documents) and considered translation tasks as common practice in FL teaching. They were all involved in the design and development of the LeViS activity taught and two of them also took the initiative to add some activities to the original lesson plan.

All LeViS sessions took place in a computer room with fewer workstations than the number of learners which meant that they worked in groups of two or three.

232 STAVROULA SOKOLI, PATRICK ZABALBEASCOA & MARIA FOUNTANA

4.2. Romania

The Romanian sample included 14 high-school learners, two girls and twelve boys, aged 15 and 16. They were all learners at the Energetic Vocational school and part of the Magyar cultural minority in Romania. Their mother tongue and the language of their regular courses is Magyar. Although Romanian is the official language, it is perceived as a foreign language to them and communication in Romanian needs continuous improvement at school.

The involvement of such young learners in pilot testing was not foreseen in the design of the questionnaires used as a tool for data collection. Consequently, some of the questions were difficult to understand and demanding since they were designed for adults. Careful consideration was therefore given to the above issues during the evaluation of data from these questionnaires.

The learners were very familiar with language learning since each one of them spoke three to four foreign languages on average (including their mother tongue). Their level of competence in the language taught was upper intermediate (B2 level). They also responded that they did computer activities in language learning classes at school and that they used computers daily outside school, mainly for playing games, chatting and doing their homework.

The teacher who taught the LeViS activity was an Information Technology teacher with a special interest in FLL and translation and was actively involved in the design and development of the activity.

The activity was taught in the Energetic Technical College in Brasov, in an IT lab with fewer workstations than the number of learners. Learners worked in pairs and sat in the same places they did for other subjects.

4.3. UK

Implementation in the UK was limited to two British learners (21 and 28 years old) and one 20-year-old student from Luxembourg who spoke five languages. They were all studying Spanish at Roehampton University.

All three learners were familiar with computer activities in FLL (word processing, e-mail and internet use) and they felt that an increase in the number of computer activities would be a positive element in their language classes. They all had the necessary IT skills to take full advantage of their computer after class. Only one of them was very familiar with translation activities as a language student but they all seemed to like the idea. They had moderate experience of using video or multimedia in FLL, which was evaluated as quite good.

The teacher was quite experienced in translation both as an FL teacher and as a freelancer. She also used AV material quite often in her lessons. She was a member of the Roehampton team that actually designed the activity.

4.4. Portugal

Implementation in Portugal was carried out in two different groups: a group of Portuguese learners of English (B2 level of competence) at the University of Algarve, and a group of Ukrainian learners of Portuguese. It was not possible to collect questionnaires from the second group because the course was intensive and there was no time to hand out the questionnaire in class.

The informants were very familiar with language learning. They did computer activities in language classes on a regular basis, and answered that they would be happy to have even more computer activities in their course. They were all quite familiar with computer use outside language classes either for learning purposes or for personal entertainment and communication with other people.

Activities involved intralingual and not interlingual subtitling, in other words, learners were asked not to translate but to transcribe the dialogues. 60% of the learners answered that they had either no or limited experience with translation as language learners and stated that they liked it somewhat* (3/5). This was also the case regarding their experience with video or multimedia as language learners.

The teacher was not against translation as a task for FLL, which she had indeed occasionally used in her teaching along with audiovisual prompts (e.g. use of video). She was a member of the development team of the activities for Portuguese learners.

4.5. Greece

The informants in Greece were Erasmus learners of Greek studying at the University of Patras. All learners were undergraduates from various countries studying civil engineering, computer engineering, geology etc. Three of them were women and five were men.

In addition, questionnaires were collected from groups who used LeViS activities for purposes other than language learning. More specifically, activities were designed for and used by a group of secondary school students in their computer science class.

All three teachers who completed the evaluation questionnaires were involved in the design of the activities and were very familiar with the use of the software.

4.6. Spain

Implementation in Spain could be said to be the most interesting in relation to both its extent and the people involved, who were teachers and students at the Translation and Interpretation Faculty of the Universitat Autònoma de Barcelona. A full description of the experience at the UAB (objectives, materials, activity description) can be found in Romero et al. (forthcoming).

Activities were used in three different language courses of Italian (C1 level), Portuguese (C1 level) and Chinese (A1 level).

All learners from the three groups had common characteristics. They had different mother tongues and most of them often did computer activities in language learning classes. The most popular computer activities included the use of e-mail, videoviewer, internet resources and spreadsheets.

40% of the learners were pretty happy* (3/5) with the number of computer activities implemented in their course, whereas 37% would rather do
more* (6/7) computer activities. Most of them also used a computer outside classes several times a week for learning purposes or communication
with other people.

As expected, almost all learners were familiar with translation as language learners and their experience was positive. Most of them responded
that they like translation as a task. Half of them had little or some experience* (2 or 3/5) using video or multimedia either as language learners
or independently of language. Most of them evaluated their experience
using video or multimedia for language learning as quite or very good*
(4 or 5/5).

All three teachers involved in the implementation phase were also
professional translators and were all involved in the development of the
activities. They also had a personal opinion deriving from their professional experience on how translation should be used in FLL, which they
considered as a useful task.

5. What learners and teachers think

A combination of qualitative and quantitative techniques (Oliver, 2000)
was used, with special emphasis on the qualitative interpretation of data.
Qualitative analysis aims to give answers to questions looking for a "how"
or a "what" (Creswell, 1998). This kind of analysis aims to produce an
understanding of processes through the study of correlations, rather than
the study of reason-result relations, which are the scope of quantitative
analysis.

Due to the limited extent of this paper, the results of the data analysis
are not presented in detail. A full account of the evaluation including charts
and percentages can be found in the project report (Fountana et al., 2008).
A synthesis of the results is presented in the following points.

5.1. About the software

Most of the learners and all teachers participating in the project consider the software to be a very or quite a useful tool* (4 or 5/5) for FL learning and teaching. They also think that it is very or quite appropriate* (4 or 5/5) for the activity they were involved in.

The main advantages of the LvS software, as reported by learners and teachers may be summarized in the following list: it is life-like and productive; it offers opportunities for creative use of language; it promotes collaborative and individual learning depending on the goals of the activities; it combines image, sound and text production; the video clips are suitable for practicing different competencies; it has an interesting interface by making use of 4 areas; it is motivating, multicultural, interdisciplinary, well-structured and entertaining but also provides the versatility to prepare different types of activities to practice different skills.

The main disadvantages of the LvS software, as reported by teachers, are that: creating and designing an activity is time-consuming; some computer skills are needed; activities are technology-dependent thus often interrupted for different reasons, such as incompatibility of resources.

Main suggestions for improving the LvS software are: add the functionality of a spell checker; optimize cueing techniques; add text formatting tools; include dictionaries; have a "comparison" tool available in order to compare the subtitles of peers, or to use two or more clips simultaneously; have a language submenu available at options menu; splitter handles and tooltips should be added describing drag and double-click actions; resizing of interface areas should be made more clear; improve the "save as" function; pay attention to multilinguality issues (e.g. have the environment available in many languages); pay attention to download and installation issues, for example, make it possible to use online so that one does not have to install it on each computer. Some of the issues identified by the informants were addressed before the project ended, including multilinguality (LvS is available in six languages), tooltips and other technical issues.

5.2. About the activities

Overall, learners judged the activities positively. A high percentage of learners found the activities very or quite interesting* (72% with 4 or 5/5), very or quite fun and entertaining* (60% with 4 or 5/5) and only a few of them thought that the activities were very or quite hard* (12% with 4 or 5/5). Significantly, most of the students expressed their wish to have more LeViS activities* (68% with 4 or 5/5) in their regular FL course.

Learners with previous experience of video and multimedia in their courses, tended to consider it positively.

All teachers would consider using LeViS activities regularly in the language learning sessions as a means of alternative teaching and learning approach, with the exception of one teacher who believes that this approach is more suitable and convenient for individual learning. All teachers would consider developing LeViS activities on their own for future use.

Other issues considered important in relation to using the software regularly in classroom are: the availability of computers; the availability of ready-made activities to choose from, as they are time-consuming to design and create; the availability of ready-made material that would permit the generation of new activities more quickly, for example, through a library of video clips available for importing.

Main suggestions for improving the LeViS activities include: develop similar questions within the activity to the ones used in class; use easier dialogues for beginners; increase the difficulty of the activities for more advanced learners; have learners do the activities both individually and in groups; increase the amount of listening and comprehension activities; decrease the duration of the activity; add more activities within the software; have video selection from cartoons and action movies; offer the alternative of working with a series even if this would imply different sessions and working individually at home or in the computer room; preparing more activities with different audiovisual genres where language is used differently; have tasks available which are less prepared by the author (for example, involve the learners in cueing the subtitles) so that students can explore all the possibilities of the software and be more autonomous.

5.3. About the approach

Teachers were worried that their learners would not cope well with technology but similar to what is indicated from the results of other projects (Egarchou et al., 2007), their learners proved them wrong.

Teachers noticed that learners' overall participation had in no case been lower than usual. On the contrary, 70% of the teachers, when asked, answered that learners' overall participation might have been higher than usual.

Half of the teachers also felt that the activities taught had achieved their goals to the full* (5/5). Three teachers thought that the goals had been achieved quite a lot* (4/5) and two that their goals had been achieved somewhat* (3/5). They reported that they used them as an icebreaker and a pleasant change, to promote differences between oral and written speech, to attract students' interest, to focus on new, contextualized structures and expressions, to develop synthesis skills, to work with different media in one platform, and to plan a range of activities, among others.

Learners and teachers are unsure whether this approach could be useful for learning subjects other than foreign languages. Many suggest that it could prove valuable in learning any lesson on culture, history, linguistics, art etc. In any case, they all agree that it should be tried out more extensively.

6. Discussion and conclusions

The timeliness of the project can be seen in other parallel developments that have taken place over the last two years. There has been a boom in the number of internet sites illustrating what the new trends in education are and where we are headed. The key words in this respect are precisely: internet, multimedia, multimodal, and multilingual. The LeViS project provides insight, proposals and materials for all of them. This impressive growth was not so easy to foresee when the LeViS project began.

One of the strengths of the LvS software is that it can hold any audio-visual format, although it requires authors or materials providers to supply clips, usually conceived of as short footage of about one to five minutes.

Another essential component of the LeViS project, subtitling, has also been affected by the technological and internet boom (Talaván Zanón, this volume). On this point, we might say that LeViS has played an active role in bringing this about. But it must also be said that the wide range of different subtitling software and environments to be found online, would probably cause the results of the questionnaires carried out during the LeViS project to change quite considerably regarding the students' and teachers' familiarity with subtitling, both as a regular form of communication (online and offline), and as a tool frequently used in FL education.

The LeViS project evaluation showed that LvS software is felt to be reliable and user-friendly as well as adequate for the purpose for which it was designed, i.e. a resource for FLL.

Important findings were made during the process of designing activities that could show prospective learners how to benefit most from the software and the LeViS concept. That is, the researchers as teachers found that while working on the project they were focusing much of their thinking on the broader context of LeViS, on crucial issues to do with what is taught, how it is taught, and how individual exercises must fit in a well-prepared lesson plan, which in turn must fit in a thoroughly thought out syllabus. The language learning approach is a product of close partner collaboration with the involvement of expert teachers. As a result, teachers who used the LvS activities for FLL think that they met their teaching goals and methods quite a lot in many different ways.

All sample activities developed follow a well structured and consistent lesson-plan format which includes information regarding the objectives and the aim of the LvS activity, the appropriate context and the estimated student profile for implementing each specific activity, a breakdown of the teaching approach describing also the teacher and student roles in each phase and finally the expected outcomes and suggestions for possible deviations from the plan.

Sample activities, where implemented extensively, provided rich teacher and student feedback including suggestions for improving the software, the methodology and the sample activities themselves.

Sample activities covered a wide variety of tasks and materials. Some video material was produced by the students themselves, and by the tutors, some materials involved role-play and acting out real-life scenarios, or simulations of them. Others were clips from feature films, television series, or short musical videos, showing that the range of possible video materials is practically limitless, and the range of possible exercises is only limited by the users' imagination and experience.

This project has also succeeded in its stated aim of providing materials, resources, and ideas for teachers of less widely-spread European languages. This is a major asset, as has already been mentioned above given the boom in online and DVD resources for FLL. However, it must be said that most of it is for English, French and German.

One of the most important findings of the evaluation was that learners of different languages, from different backgrounds and at different levels felt they benefited from being involved in subtitling activities and consider LvS a useful tool. In particular, they showed their feelings by expressing a keen interest in spending more classroom time doing subtitling activities. Their interest and high motivation was also evidenced in their participation as reported by teachers.

We are confident that this project and its by-products and side effects will live on in the future and will appear in the literature as a milestone for distance learning and FL teaching methods and approaches for a long time to come.

As we move closer towards a Society of Technology and Communication, as universities become more adapted to certain initiatives (e.g. the Common European Framework, the European portfolio for languages, the Bologna Process), students and tutors alike will become more familiar with the tools and the right frame of mind to get the most out of thinking in terms of multimodality and computer technology in combination with well-based imaginative approaches to FL teaching, and multilingualism.

References

Allan, M. (1985), *Teaching English with Video*. London: Longman.

BECTA (2004), What the Research Says about Using ICT in Modern Foreign Languages, Coventry, BECTA: <http://research.becta.org.uk/upload-dir/downloads/page_documents/research/wtrs_mfl.pdf> (accessed 17/06/2010).

Borrás, I., and R. C. Lafayette (1994), Effects of Multimedia Courseware Subtitling on the Speaking Performance of College Learners of French. *Modern Language Journal* 78(1), 61–75.

Ciccone, A. (1995), Teaching with Authentic Video: Theory and Practice. In F. R. Eckman, D. Highland, P. W. Lee, J. Mileham and R. Rutkowski (eds), *Second Language Acquisition Theory and Pedagogy*. New Jersey, Hove: Lawrence Erlbaum Associates, 203–16.

Creswell, J. W. (1998), *Qualitative Inquiry and Research Design: Choosing among Five Traditions*. London: Sage Publications.

Danan, M. (1992), Reversed Subtitling and Dual Coding Theory: New Directions for Foreign Language Instruction. *Language Learning* 42(4), 497–527.

Egarchou, D., M. Fountana, C. Roniotes, T. Hadzilacos and N. Sifakis (2007), What We Have Learned from the Implementation of the Mustlearnit Project: The Greek Point of View and Experience. In proceedings of the MustLearnIT Conference, Syros, Greece, 20–22 September, 1–15.

Fountana, M., and D. Egarchou (2008), *ICT Expert Evaluation Report*. <http://levis.cti.gr> Document Library, file name D6.1a_Expert_Evaluation_Report_v.1.0.doc (accessed 17/06/2010).

Gambier, Y. (2007), Sous-titrage et apprentissage des langues. *Linguistica Antwerpiensia* 6, 97–113.

King, J. (2002), Using DVD Feature Films in the EFL Classroom. *Computer Assisted Language Learning* 15, 509–23.

Klerkx, J. (1998), The Place of Subtitling in a Translator Training Course. *Teaching Translation in Universities. Present and Future Perspectives*. London: CILT, 259–64.

Kostaras, N., D. Stavrinoudis, S. Sokoli and M. Xenos (2010), Combining Experimental and Inquiry Methods in Software Usability Evaluation: The Paradigm of Lvs Educational Software. *Journal of Systems and Information Technology* 12(2), 120–39.

Neves, J. (2004), Language Awareness Through Training in Subtitling. In P. Orero (ed.), *Topics in Audiovisual Translation*. Amsterdam: John Benjamins, 127–40.

Oliver, M. (2000), An Introduction to the Evaluation of Learning Technology. *Educational Technology & Society* 3(4), 20–30.

Romero, L., O. Torres and S. Sokoli (forthcoming), La subtitulación al servicio del aprendizaje de lenguas para traductores: el entorno LvS, *Babel: Revue internationale de la traduction*.

Sokoli, S. (2006), Learning via Subtitling (LvS): A Tool for the Creation of Foreign Language Learning Activities Based on Film Subtitling. In M. Carroll and H. Gerzymisch-Arbogast (eds), *Audiovisual Translation Scenarios: Proceedings of the Marie Curie Euroconferences*.

Stempleski, S., and B. Tomalin (1990), *Video in Action: Recipes for Using Video in Language Teaching*. London: Prentice Hall.

Tomalin, B. (1990), *Video in the English Class. Techniques for Successful Teaching*. BBC English.

Tschirner, E. (2001), Language Acquisition in the Classroom: The Role of Digital Video. *Computer Assisted Language Learning* 14(3–4), 305–19.

Williams, H., and D. Thorne (2000), The Value of Teletext Subtitling as a Medium for Language Learning, *System* 28(2), 217–28.

Zabalbeascoa, P. (2010), Translation in Constrained Communication and Entertainment. In J. Díaz-Cintas, A. Matamala and J. Neves (eds), *New Insights into Audiovisual Translation and Media Accessibility*. Amsterdam: Rodopi, 25–40.

LAURA INCALCATERRA MCLOUGHLIN AND JENNIFER LERTOLA

Learn through Subtitling:
Subtitling as an Aid to Language Learning

1. Theoretical framework

This article presents a theoretical framework for using film subtitling in foreign language classes and suggests a detailed structure for its integration in the foreign language (FL) syllabus. We propose a practical subtitling activity with a lesson plan which follows a five-phase model: motivation, global comprehension, analysis, synthesis and reflection.

The utilization of subtitled material in FL classes is widespread and several international studies have confirmed the validity of such an approach particularly in relation to listening, reading and speaking skills. However, literature on the integration of subtitling in FL curricula and its effectiveness is perhaps less extensive, even though there is considerable interest in this area (Bravo, 2008; Díaz-Cíntas, 2001; Neves, 2004; Talaván Zanón, 2006, this volume). Indeed the realization of the LeVis[1] platform has certainly gone a long way in facilitating tutors who wish to introduce this challenging but rewarding activity (Sokoli et al., this volume).

A number of reasons can be cited to support the creation of subtitles in FL classes: it facilitates mnemonic retention and language awareness (including pragmatic awareness), it lends itself to collaborative projects, generates emotionally charged activities which keep learners motivated, it is innovative and fun. Subtitling activities also promote learner's autonomy as learners observe communication acts and advance hypotheses on how to

---

[1]   LeVis: <http://levis.cti.gr/> (accessed 3/11/2010).

interpret them. However, subtitling is ultimately a translation exercise. So, what makes it so different from written, textual translations which, with varied fortunes, have traditionally been used in FL teaching?

Apart from obvious considerations on the polysemiotic nature of a filmic text, and apart from the contextualization of verbal communication within a realistic environment, the translation element of subtitling implies linguistic and meta-linguistic awareness as well as an ability for contrastive analysis, skills which are also necessary in order to complete a monosemiotic, written translation task. However, when written translations are incorporated in FL teaching, they are often closed, self-referential systems which exclude the wider linguistic universe that students must grasp, when operating in a foreign language. This does not deny the validity of the use of translation in FL teaching; indeed after a period of adverse favour during the latter part of the last century, more recent studies have reaffirmed its value. Atkinson (1987: 243) indicated that it is students' "preferred strategy [and] an inevitable part of second language acquisition" and indeed research suggests that translation is an effective cognitive strategy for learning foreign vocabulary. So the challenge is to move from a closed, self-referential system to one where there is scope for a wider communicational context, in which the verbal element of the communicative act in FL is reinforced and complemented by the non-verbal elements which add meaning to each utterance. Many texts lend themselves well to this purpose, particularly – but not exclusively – certain audiovisual texts (films, TV series, soap operas etc). Audiovisual translation has the added bonus of making it immediately evident that there is a communicative reason for the translation (rather than a grammatical reason, for example), thereby according a meaningful functional dimension to the new TL text. In relation to language learning, as well as assisting enhanced listening skills, vocabulary building and retention and intercultural awareness, subtitling can also lead to the acquisition of linguistic structures because of its laborious and repetitive nature: learners who are able to manipulate input (literally, through typing, synchronizing, trial and error tasks on their keyboards) are processing information holistically and are therefore in a position to memorize structures without necessarily being consciously aware of it.[2]

Before moving on to the presentation of the proposed activity, we must stress that the purpose is not to train professional subtitlers; for this reason the technical parameters are not always observed to the letter. As for the refinement of skills related to translation, whilst it may constitute a desirable consequence of the didactic journey, it is not pursued systematically here, as it is felt that it should rather be included among the objectives for higher levels of fluency (at least B2, but possibly higher).

1.1. Technical aspects of subtitling

The technical aspects of subtitling represent a constraining factor limiting translators' freedom by forcing them to revise the message of the ST and adopt concise solutions which, being immediately receptive to the viewer, are otherwise faithful – where possible – to the pragmalinguistic specificity of the ST. Film subtitles are generally limited to a maximum of some 40 characters (spaces included) per line, extending for not more than two lines and remaining on the screen for a duration ranging from one to six seconds approximately. Subtitles remaining visible for a period longer than six seconds tend to be read more than once by the viewer, altering the continuity and flow of speech. In Western countries they are normally placed at the bottom of the screen, centred or left aligned.

2 During trials, the authors found high levels of retention of linguistic structures: 68% of noun phrases and 88% of verb phrases were retained two weeks after subtitling, although more research is needed to subtantiate further these findings.

2. Methods and procedures

The activity was tested on classes of intermediate level (B1) at the School of Languages, Literatures & Cultures (Italian Studies), National University of Ireland, Galway, during the academic year 2008–9. However, the activity may be changed and adapted for use with lower (A2) or higher levels (B2–C2).

2.1. Selection of material

While activities may be designed for the subtitling of films, documentaries, news bulletins, advertising or other types of video clips, consistent with the needs and interests of recipients, we would recommend the use of authentic video material – not dubbed from another language or created for educational purposes – in order to provide learners with a realistic language experience.[3] In choosing video material, it will be necessary to consider the:

- needs and motivations of learners;
- linguistic complexity of the material in relation to the competence level of learners;
- previous linguistic and cultural knowledge of learners;
- paralinguistic and extra-linguistic content of material;
- length of the material.[4]

---

3   We refer to authentic material in the sense also used, among others, by Garza (1996) and Omaggio-Hadley (2001), i.e. material created for use by native speakers and therefore devoid of didactic purposes.

4   According to the Common European Framework of Reference (CEFR), when selecting texts (whether oral or written), various factors should be considered: linguistic complexity, text type, length, discursive structure, the channels through which the text is presented, the interest the text has for the learner (CEFR, 2001: 201–2).

In this instance, we opted for a film, because: "thanks to the authenticity of films we can enter into a culture, into the way people live, dress, eat, relate. The film is a window opening onto a culture that allows us to make contact and understand its values" (Convertini, 2006: 22, our translation). In particular, the film *Manuale d'amore* by Giovanni Veronesi (2005) was chosen for the following reasons: the protagonists are peers of our students, the situation in question can adapt well to their interests and experiences, and the setting, in Rome, provides numerous opportunities for sociocultural and intercultural comparison and reflection.

The narrative structure of *Manuale d'amore* is another important reason for our film choice. The division into self-contained episodes renders its use for didactic purposes particularly easy as students can be presented with a short story which is, nonetheless, complete and well developed. However, the scene to be subtitled should be much shorter than a whole episode, between three and five minutes (in the case of the course held at the National University of Ireland the episode lasted 3'10").

2.2. Preparation and phases of activity

The activity requires the availability of the following tools:

- video material in a format compatible with the software for subtitling (generally *.wmv, .mpg, .avi*);
- screen (or TV) and DVD player for watching the video;
- PCs / laptops with DVD player, word processor (*Word* or *Notepad*) and subtitling software (at least one PC / laptop for every 3 students);
- video-editing software (available to the teacher);
- black / white board;
- transcript of the scene to be subtitled.

A range of freely downloadable subtitling software is available, however, we found *DivXLand Media Subtitler* to be a good, user-friendly solution.[5] *Windows Movie Maker* can be used for video-editing.[6]

The work in class is divided into five phases and follows a preparatory stage, involving only the teacher, which consists of:

1. Selection and preparation of the material to be viewed and subtitled (i.e. the choice of video and scene to present to the class);
2. Transcription of verbal content (or, if possible, sourcing of a version on the internet). The transcript must submit each line of dialogue on a line to itself, therefore there will be a full stop at the end of each line of dialogue;
3. Familiarization with the subtitling program.

Work in class is divided into a first phase necessarily devoted to motivation – which includes an overview of the subtitles and their technical characteristics (section 1.1.) – and four further phases: globality, analysis, synthesis and reflection.

Malakoff and Hakuta (1991: 149) describe translation as linguistic manipulation operating on a dual level: understanding the message in the original and developing an appropriate phrasal structure in the target language in which to capture that message. Four semantic-linguistic processes are intertwined with these two levels: "understanding of the vocabulary of the source text, understanding of the meaning of the message in the source

---

5   *DivXLand Media Subtitler* can be dowloaded freely from <http://www.divxland. org> (accessed 3/11/2010). The site provides information about video formats compatible with DivXLand. The software is extremely easy to use and requires no special computer skills. Other free and easy-to-use programs are also available. In particular, *Subtitle Workshop* (downloadable from <http://www.urusoft.net>; accessed 3/11/2010) offers linear and intuitive solutions and is an excellent alternative to the software used here.

6   *Windows Movie Maker* is generally present in every computer using the *Windows* operating system; it is downloadable free of charge from <http://www.microsoft. com> (accessed 3/11/2010). This program allows users to cut video files with extreme ease.

language, reformulation of the message in the target language, reflection on the adequacy of the target text" (ibid.), where reformulation and reflection, the authors specify, are applied both on the level of structure and meaning. The division into phases of the learning activity proposed here was devised taking into consideration this complex system of linguistic-textual processing; therefore, after motivation, the globality and analysis phases will cover the first two processes listed by Malakoff and Hakuta, whilst synthesis and reflection are linked to the last two.

Table 25 summarizes the organization of our teaching activity in chart form:

Table 25: Outline of teaching activities

Phase of activity	Objectives	Material	Execution
Preparation (exclusively for teachers) Duration: 2–3 hrs	Preparation of material. Familiarization with software to be used.	Video (DVD or other formats). *Windows Movie Maker* (or similar).	Selection and preparation of materials for subtitling. Transcription of the dialogue.
Motivation Duration: 45 mins	Creation of motivation. Emotional involvement. Creation / reinforcement of group cohesion.	Black / white board. Internet (if available).	Presentation of activity. Overview of subtitling. Formulation of hypotheses on chosen video.
Globality Duration: 45 mins	Global comprehension. Formulate and present hypotheses.	TV / PC / screen with DVD player.	Viewing of the scene. Group discussion. Viewing with transcription.

Analysis Duration: 45 mins	Analytical comprehension. Develop awareness of linguistic, pragma- and paralinguistic elements of communication.	PCs / laptops. Word processor (*Microsoft Word, Notepad, Open OfficeWriter etc.*).	Discussion on linguistic and paralinguistic aspects of the message and their interpretation.
Synthesis Duration: 2–3 hrs	Reformulation of message in form of subtitles in TL.	PCs/laptops Subtitling software (*DivXLand* or similar).	Translation, subtitling and synchronization of the scene.
Reflection Duration: 45 mins	Reflection on adequacy of subtitles. Develop self-criticism and self-correction.	Blackboard PCs/laptops Subtitling software (*DivXLand* or similar).	Viewing subtitled scene. Corrections and final editing.

2.3. Motivation

The motivation phase is a necessary starting point, but the teacher must naturally maintain and reinforce motivation during the entire course of the teaching activity. This is even more important during subtitling because technical difficulties are added to linguistic difficulties. Initially, it will be necessary to work on motivation by selecting video material that corresponds to the learners' interests – in order to stimulate emotional involvement – and to underline the immediate communicative usability of the task.

During this initial phase, the teacher will endeavour to create a working environment in which students can interact informally, thus avoiding states of anxiety due to both the linguistic input and the technological tools; the playful aspect of the activity should be emphasized, rather than its technical characteristics. To begin, the teacher:

1. explains the activity to students, encouraging them to become more aware of and responsible for their own learning. S/he also provides an overview of the technical and theoretical aspects of subtitling. In particular, it should be noted that this process involves the transition from spoken to written code, in which the prosodic and other characteristics of the spoken code (emphasis, iteration, change of register, use of dialect forms etc.) are difficult to integrate. During analysis and synthesis students must reflect on these difficulties and propose appropriate solutions;

2. introduces the material to be subtitled and asks students to reflect on what that title suggests to them, in order to elicit past linguistic-cultural knowledge and enable "expectancy grammar". The teacher asks the students to enunciate the images, feelings and ideas, the title evokes for them and their expectations. It is advisable to write the students' responses on the board;

3. invites students to search the internet for the movie poster (in the event that a network connection is not available, the teacher can provide a photocopy of the document) to proceed with an initial examination of the hypotheses previously made and noted, in order to stimulate conversation and reinforce the cohesion of the group.

2.4. Globality

In this phase students are exposed to linguistic input in a unitary (global) way as they would in authentic communicative situations, without any intervention by the teacher before or during viewing.

The selected scene is presented in its original language. After a first run, students are invited to relate what they understood of the scene. It is advisable to allow the class to discuss freely – without intervening – and instead re-propose the viewing several times more if necessary. Comparison among peers is extremely useful because, if the majority of students have understood or guessed what was happening in the scene, each one will have grasped different details and can therefore make a contribution to the group.

The teacher then provides a transcript of the dialogue exchanges[7] and proposes a further viewing of the film clip. The scene will be watched with greater awareness as students are now motivated by the desire to identify the details noticed by their peers and find new elements to increase understanding and, in return, fuel group discussion.

The clip from *Manuale d'amore* examined here has been jokingly renamed by the authors as "Scene of the black cat" and is rich in linguistic, paralinguistic and extra-linguistic content: Tommaso, the protagonist, undergoes two unsuccessful job interviews and, while returning home on a Vespa, sees a black cat crossing the road. Already in a bad mood, he argues with a girl who seems to have stopped to avoid the cat, but her friend intervenes and Tommaso falls madly in love with her.

The scene has different linguistic registers (formal in the job interviews and informal in the meeting with the girls) and depicts speakers who differ in age, gender and accent. Tommaso speaks with a marked Roman accent, which helps to provide a taste of regional linguistic varieties and can be a starting point for further investigation. The most important extralinguistic element is linked to the superstitious belief, still valid in Italy, of the black cat as the bearer of bad luck.[8] Since certain cultural elements may be completely unknown to students, it is therefore important that the teacher verifies the full understanding of the cultural connotation of the material. In our particular case, the centrality of the cat in the meeting with the two girls must be noted and students should be invited to formulate hypotheses regarding its significance.

---

7   It is not always easy to find the screenplay of the film, so the teacher may need to transcribe the lines of dialogue. For Italian screenplays, some unpublished, see <http://www.sceneggiatori.com/scripts/index.asp> (accessed 7/11/2010).

8   The belief that black cats bring bad luck has its origin in the Middle Ages when cats, especially black ones, were associated with witchcraft. At night, one can only see a black cat's eyes, which, when reflecting the surrounding light, appear to glow in the dark. In the Middle Ages this phenomenon was thought to be caused by the devil's incarnation in the cat (Filograsso and Travaglini, 2007: 56).

2.5. Analysis

We now move on to a more in-depth analysis of the dialogue. In this phase, learners focus in greater detail on the linguistic and paralinguistic input and arrive at a greater understanding of the overall message. Teacher's intervention may be necessary, at times, to clarify doubts and direct interpretations. In this phase students:

1. identify (individually or in pairs) the idiomatic and colloquial expressions contained in the ST and try to interpret them based on their linguistic and cultural knowledge and in accordance with the context of the scene;
2. notice, with the help of the teacher, gestures, tone of voice, spatiality and other non-verbal elements that contribute to the communication of the message;
3. discuss their interpretation with classmates while the teacher facilitates understanding where dictionaries or other reference materials do not help;
4. take notes (the notes made in this phase will prove crucial later on).

From a linguistic point of view, this scene presents words and expressions which may be difficult to interpret and on which it is useful to dwell during analysis. For example, Tommaso, in his inner monologue, uses expressions such as *in piena statistica* [dead average] and *senza una lira* [pennyless]. Further colloquial expressions are: *una roba mai vista* [never saw anything like it], *hai beccato la giornatina sbagliata* [you picked the wrong day], and the ironic *allora, signorino!* [well, Sir!]. Students should advance hypotheses and discuss the meaning of these messages and then, in the next phase, identify in their own language, expressions they deem to be equivalent in register, irony, humour and so on.

2.6. Synthesis

In this phase, students proceed to translating and subtitling the scene.

If the translation focuses primarily on the verbal text of the dialogue, students cannot overlook the non-verbal elements of communication, including, in particular, the paralinguistic and extra-linguistic components. Paralinguistic elements include intonation, pronunciation, pauses and rhythm. Extra-linguistic elements include kinesics (gestures and facial expression), proxemics (the distance between the interlocutors), as well as the social significance of objects and clothes. All these aspects can influence translation choices and require the use of "verbal acrobatics" (Pavesi, 2005: 17, our translation) in order to render the target message correctly and in a comprehensible manner.

Subtitling, because of its intersemiotic nature, involves a reworking of the source language, which abandons the oral form and assumes a written one in the TT;[9] this, however, must be aligned with images and sounds as much as the original spoken text (ibid.: 39). Furthermore, in subtitling it is necessary to recognize that reading times should be minimized in order to avoid compromising simultaneous fruition of images. It should also be noted that reading of the subtitle is different from that of any other type of text: viewers are inclined to consider each individual subtitle as an independent unit, which appears only for a short time, preventing forward and backward eye movements in search of textual coherence and cohesion (Mason, 2001: 20). In this phase, students strive consider all these factors and refer to very specific strategies (Gottlieb, 1992; Diadori, 2003; Perego, 2005: 101–2). Work is ideally organized in pairs or in small groups and proceeds as follows:

---

9   For a reflection on simulated orality of film language, see Chaume (2001) and Pavesi (2005).

1. Translation of the transcript (in *Word* or *Notepad*, for example). The structure of the translation must be similar to that of the transcript (so that each remark is a line in itself) and must not contain the speaker's name. The final translation will be saved as a file with the extension *.txt* (for example: *Translation.txt*);

2. Subtitling:

    (a) Open the program *DivXLand Media Subtitler* and import the preselected video by clicking on *File → Open video* in the drop-down menu;

    (b) Import the translation created in (1) above: from the dropdown menu, simply select *File → Open Text* or *Subtitle*. The translated text will appear on the left of the screen, line by line as it was saved in the *.txt* file. It will become immediately evident that some sentences are too long and must be abbreviated, subdivided, etc.;

    (c) Note that in the *Start* and *End* columns, the value is zero, because subtitles have not yet been synchronized, i.e. no start/end times have been indicated. To start the video, select *Preview Only* (under *Captioning Mode*) and click on the start arrow. It can now be pointed out to students how speech time flows and their attention may be directed to the bar at the bottom of the video where the passing seconds are visible.

3. Subtitle synchronization. This is the most laborious part, but after a little practice students should be able to proceed smoothly. For synchronization, proceed as follows:

    (a) Click *Press* and *Hold* under *Captioning Mode* (Figure 5);

    (b) Start the video from the start arrow;

    (c) Click *Apply* at the precise moment you want the subtitle to appear (i.e. when the character begins to utter the line of dialogue) and keep it clicked for as long as you want to keep the subtitle (i.e. until the character ends the line of dialogue);

    (d) Repeat for each subtitle. The start and end times of each subtitle will now appear in the relevant columns;

    (e) To correct the times manually, click on the line of dialogue to edit and change the start time (*Show*) or duration (*Duration*) of the subtitle, as required;

(f) To correct the text of a line of dialogue (*Caption*), highlight it and make modifications in the box below, where the text of the caption appears (Figure 5) or click *Edit* and then select *Edit* again in the drop-down menu;

(g) To add a space line and insert a new line of dialogue, click *Edit* and then select *Add* in the drop-down menu. This will be useful for breaking up lines of dialogue that are too long to appear on the screen;

(h) Save the work by clicking *File* and then *Save As* from the drop-down menu. Among the file-type options, select *Substation Alpha SSA*, which will save the subtitles and the times. Whenever you want to return to working on this scene simply reopen the *.ssa* file.[10] This will not embed the subtitles into the video: video and subtitles will remain in two separate files;[11]

(i) View the work completed: *Open DivXLand*, select the *.ssa* file, the video, click *Preview Only* then the start arrow. It is only possible to view the work within DivXLand.

During this phase, students are asked to make choices in relation to translation and adaptation (synchronizing subtitles in accordance with the space-time parameters listed in section 1.1.). When the subtitled scene is viewed, the adequacy or inadequacy of the choices made is usually quite obvious. The objective here, however, is not to create the perfect subtitle, but to raise awareness of the elements which assist and facilitate linguistic communication: pragmatics, prosody, proxemics, as well as redundant features, which may need to be reduced or deleted in subtitling. Another important objective is to encourage reflection on contrastive or equivalent features pertaining to L1 and L2. This will lead students to "notice" the (foreign) language, internalizing its structures and expressions.

10   Open *DivXLand Media Subtitler*, import the video as shown in 2 *(a)* and the file *.ssa* by clicking on *File* → *Open Text* or *Subtitle* as in 2 *(b)*.

11   It is, however, possible, by downloading the necessary *codecs*, to embed subtitles on a DVD. For more information refer to <http://www.divxland.org>.

Figure 5: DivXLand Media Subtitler. Reproduced with permission.

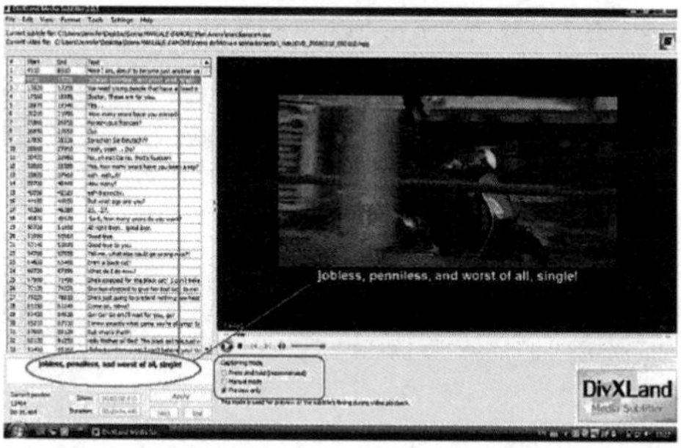

Note: It is possible to edit the text of the subtitles in the box (bottom left). Under *Captioning Mode* it is possible to synchronize (by selecting Press and Hold) or view the work in progress (by selecting *Preview only*).

Interestingly, apparently "simple" utterances tend to give rise to stimulating and pertinent discussions when students must take responsibility for translation choices that will clearly influence the subtitled film. In the case of the "Scene of the black cat", for example, the protagonist uses, albeit briefly, languages other than Italian: English, French and German. Students should think about how (and if) to render these parts of the dialogue in their own language and then check the comic effect of their solution.

The scene also includes a certain amount of foul language, which helps define Tommaso's mood. Always a delicate topic in class, given the degree of embarrassment that it may create for both teacher and learners, foul language is a linguistic reality nonetheless, and not a negligible one. Videos can be a very useful tool to deal with the issue. In this case, students must decide whether to transpose the expressions into the target language, lower their tone or censure the text. Apart from the solutions adopted, which may vary from class to class, and apart from translational adequacy, discussion of these aspects promotes awareness of the linguistic register used in the ST and its correspondence or otherwise to that used in the TT.

Proper names may also be the subject of debate: will students opt in favour of domestication or foreignization? In our film, for example, the black cat is called *Briciola* [crumb]. Will students deem it appropriate to conserve the Italian name, or will they find one in their own language? In our case, students preferred domestication and renamed the cat *Biscuits*, maintaining a certain resemblance on both phonetic and semantic levels. We would suggest that teachers leave students free to make their own translation choices, reminding them that they must be justified and defended in the final reflection phase.

2.7. Reflection

With the work of subtitling and synchronization completed, the activity ends with a reflection phase, structured as follows:

1. viewing of the subtitled scene;
2. verification of the adequacy of the translation in relation to the ST;
3. verification of the adequacy of subtitling (length of subtitles, time on the screen etc.). If necessary, at this stage, a final editing can be made;
4. final discussion on the translation choices made and on the completed product.

3. Additional activities

The subtitling tasks presented here were supported by additional activities aimed at achieving greater cooperation among students. They were based on the use of *wiki*[12] and *forum* which, in our case, were available within the VLE – virtual learning environment – Blackboard platform. Students were encouraged to publish their subtitled dialogue on *wiki* in order to

---

12   *Wiki* is a collaborative piece of software, which allows for the creation of collaborative texts: users of *wiki* can add, edit or even delete what other users have inserted.

make it available to all their peers, who could then intervene by modifying or correcting it, as they deemed necessary.

The *forum* was used to communicate the changes and additions made and to discuss possible doubts or translation difficulties as well as any other matter pertaining to the project. While a *wiki* is generally only available within multimedia platforms, *forum* and *blog* necessitate only an internet connection and can be easily created without the need for specific technical skills.[13]

4. Our experience

4.1. Reflections and suggestions

The realization of this classroom activity was a positive experience, which students found innovative, fun and useful for both language learning and for a greater understanding of the pragmatic and extra-linguistic mechanisms of communication. In particular, students stressed that they were happy with the level of understanding reached during exposure to the colloquial expressions used by native peers (the actors).[14]

A positive side-effect was the level of cohesion achieved in class during this project, as well as the acquisition of technical transferable skills. In this regard, group or pair work is certainly preferable, as it helps to transform technical and linguistic difficulties into "fun" challenges and, by increasing learners' emotional involvement, strengthens motivation.

In order to optimize the results obtainable with subtitling it is advisable to plan a minimum of two teaching activities. Translation, adaptation

---

13 Many sites allow easy and intuitive creation of blogs, among them: <http://www.blogger.com> and <http://www.blogattivo.com> (both accessed 3/11/2010).

14 Students expressed their opinions in a reflective essay at the end of the first semester of the academic year 2008–9.

and (relative) synchronization require a degree of familiarity that can only be acquired through practice. Following subtitling a number of different clips, it will be noticed how greater mastery of technical means and finer understanding of subtitling strategies lead to a greater degree of "boldness" in researching and proposing translation solutions appropriate to the context.

All teaching activities included in the course offered at the National University of Ireland were accompanied by activities for reflection and exchange of ideas on *wiki* and *forum*. Not all students were actively involved in this phase, which took place outside contact hours. Those who participated found the collaboration useful, but some considered this extra time as superfluous, given that there was also an opportunity for debate and class discussion. These additional tools certainly have several advantages: *wiki*, *forum* and *blog* make it possible for students to work asynchronously, overcome "shyness", participate from anywhere at any time and reflect individually on the work done in class. We would suggest that, if these additional resources are to be used, it is important to clearly outline their purpose and benefits – in terms of learning – at the beginning of the activity, at the motivation stage, and spend some time in class reviewing and evaluating collectively the results of this collaboration online. If available, a *chat* can also be used profitably. This communication environment naturally requires that students are connected at the same time, and for this reason, may be less effective than other electronic media; however, due to its synchronous nature, it tends to facilitate and speed up work, facilitating an immediate exchange of ideas.

One incentive that played a large part in the project's success and contributed significantly to maintaining motivation during the twenty-four weeks of the course was the prospect of creating a short subtitled video to be shown to other students. The participants applied themselves assiduously, even working overtime during the final weeks in order to achieve this objective, and were rewarded by a positive reception by other students of the National University of Ireland. This final objective, dedicated to the sharing of the work done, prompted students to think about subtitles in relation to recipients and added a functional perspective to the skills developed.

4.2. Possible variations

Subtitling can also be used in the context of microlanguages, by choosing text types of specific interest. Within a specialist language course, it can represent a stimulating diversion as well as an innovative method for memorizing vocabulary and structures and integrating cultural information. In this context, documentaries, specialist bulletins (economic, scientific etc.), corporate videos, and commercials can be selected.

The creation of subtitles can also be introduced at levels of linguistic proficiency higher than those considered here. However, in such a case – and especially with learners at C1 and C2 levels – more time should be dedicated to reflection on the characteristics of subtitles and applicable strategies. The objectives of the activity may also require modification in order to place less emphasis on learning and memorizing, but probably more on refinement of translation skills, understanding of the translation process etc.

Finding suitable video material is not always easy but some internet sites provide the possibility of downloading copyright-free video material (see under References). The majority of the material is in English and, unfortunately, dated. However, with a little patience, it is possible to find suitable material suitable even in languages other than English.

References

Atkinson, D. (1987), The Mother Tongue in the Classroom: A Neglected Resource? *ELT Journal* 41(4), 241–7.
Balboni, P. (2002), *Le sfide di Babele. Insegnare le lingue nelle società complesse*. Torino: UTET Libreria.
Bardovi-Harlig, K., and Z. Dörney (1998), Language Learners Recognize Pragmatic Violations? Pragmatic Versus Grammatical Awareness in Instructed L2 Learning. *TESOL Quarterly* 32(2), 233–62.

Borrás, I., and R. Lafayette (1994), Effects of Multimedia Courseware Subtitling on the Speaking Performance of College Students of French. *The Modern Language Journal* 78(1), 61–75.

Bravo, M. C. (2008), *Putting the Reader in the Picture: Screen Translation and Foreign-Language Learning*, Doctoral Thesis. Tarragona: Universitat Rovira I Virgili.

Cardona, M. (ed.) (2007), *Vedere per capire e parlare. Il testo audiovisivo nella didattica delle lingue*. Torino: UTET Università.

Chaume, F. (2001), La pretendida oralidad de los textos audiovisuales y sus implicaciones en traducción. In F. Chaume and R. Agost (eds), *La traducción en los medios audiovisuales*. Castelló: Publicacions de la Universitat Jaume I, 77–87.

Convertini, T. (2006), Insegnare lingua con il cinema: una prospettiva alternativa. *Italica* 83(1), 22–33.

Council of Europe (2001), *Common European Framework of Reference for Languages: Learning, Teaching, Assessment*. Cambridge: Cambridge University Press.

Diadori, P. (ed.) (2001), *Insegnare italiano a stranieri*. Firenze: Le Monnier.

——(2003), Doppiaggio, sottotitoli e fenomeni di code-switching e code-mixing: la traduzione dei testi mistilingui. *Italica* 80(4), 531–41.

Díaz Cintas, J. (2001), Teaching Subtitling at University. In S. Cunico (ed.), *Training Translators and Interpreters in the New Millennium*. Portsmouth: University of Portsmouth, 29–44.

Faber, P. (1998), Translation Competence and Language Awareness. *Language Awareness* 7(1), 9–21.

Filograsso, N., and R. Travaglini (2007), *Piaget e l'educazione della mente*. Milano: Franco Angeli.

Garza, T. J. (1991), Evaluating the Use of Captioned Video Materials in Advanced Foreign Language Learning. *Foreign Language Annals* 24(3), 239–59.

——(1996), The Message is the Medium: Using Video Materials to Facilitate Foreign Language Performance. *Texas Papers in Foreign Language Education* 2, 1–18.

——and Gottlieb, H. (1992), Subtitling. A New University Discipline. In C. Dollerup and A. Loddegaard (eds), *Teaching Translation and Interpreting. Training, Talent and Experience*. Amsterdam: John Benjamins, 161–70.

Kirsten M. H. (2010), Translation and Short-Term L2 Vocabulary Retention: Hindrance or Help? *Language Teaching Research* 14(1), 61–74.

Malakoff, M., and K. Hakuta (1991), Translation Skill and Metalinguistic Awareness. In E. Bialystok (ed.), *Language Processing in Bilingual Children*. Cambridge: Cambridge University Press, 141–66.

Mason, I. (2001), Coherence in Subtitling: The Negotiation of Face. In F. Chaume and R. Agost (eds), *La traducción en los medios audiovisuales*. Castelló: Publicacions de la Universitat Jaume I, 19–31.

Neves, J. (2004), Language Awareness through Training in Subtitling. In P. Orero (ed.), *Topics in Audiovisual Translation*. Amsterdam: John Benjamins, 127–39.

Omaggio-Hadley, A. (2001), *Teaching Language in Context*. Boston: Heinle & Heinle.

Paivio, A. (1969), Mental Imagery in Associative Learning and Memory. *Psychological Review* 76(3), 241–63.

—— (1986), *Mental Representations: A Dual Coding Approach*. Oxford: Oxford University Press.

Pavesi, M. (2005), *La traduzione filmica. Aspetti del parlato dall'inglese all'italiano*. Roma: Carocci.

Perego, E. (2005), *La traduzione audiovisiva*. Roma: Carocci.

Picchiassi, M. (2007), *Apprendere l'italiano L2 nell'era digitale*. Perugia: Guerra.

Price, K. (1983), Closed-Captioned TV: An Untapped Resource. *MATSOL Newsletter* 12(2), 1–8.

Sokoli, S. (2006), Learning via Subtitling (LvS). A Tool for the Creation of Foreign Language Learning Activities Based on Film Subtitling. In M. Carroll, H. Gerzymisch-Arbogast and S. Nauert (eds), *Multidimensional Translation: Audiovisual Translation Scenarios*. Copenhagen: Advanced Translation Research Center (ATRC), 66–73.

Talaván Zanón, N. (2006), Using Subtitles to Enhance Foreign Language Learning. *Porta linguarum* 6, 41–52.

Williams, H., and D. Thorne (2000), The Value of Teletext Subtitling as a Medium for Language Learning. *System* 28, 218–28.

CARLO EUGENI

A Professional's Perspective

Could you outline how a subtitler's work is organized? Does work for DVD and TV subtitles or for interlingual and intralingual subtitles differ significantly?

A subtitler's work is far from being organized. Far too often, one receives the file to be subtitled later than is desirable in order to do a good job. However, the processes of interlingual and intralingual subtitling are more or less similar.

First step: reception of file to "translate". It may be the dialogue list only, the video only, or both the dialogue list and the video. Difficulties related to receiving only one document are self-evident.

Second step: an overview of the file(s) in order to understand textual structure and register, the main characters, the plot etc.

Third step: interlingual or intralingual translation of the text.

Fourth step: review of the finished product. If there are very strict time deadlines, more than one subtitler may work on the same file, especially if it is very long. In this case, the reviewer must endeavour to produce a consistent and coherent final text. Then the subtitles are saved as a separate file, or burnt onto the video (if requested), and the final product is sent to the client.

Producing DVD subtitles is not that different from producing TV subtitles. Upon reception of the file(s), it is necessary to verify whether there are particular conventions that should be followed. If not, in-house conventions are adopted. Then the work is carried out as described above. However, one difference between subtitling for DVD or TV lies in deadlines and in the distribution of the work. The DVD market is happier to tolerate delays than television, where a programme must go on air at a given time and subtitles must be received in advance of that time. It is not unusual, when working for TV, that a file is received just hours before a programme is due to be broadcast and thus there is very little time to work on an adequate translation and to review it accurately. It sometimes occurs that a subtitling file is ready and sent to the broadcaster just minutes before the programme goes on air.

TV subtitling is generally simpler than DVD subtitling. The former is generally undertaken by an external company or by the broadcaster's own subtitling service and the same subtitler goes through all aforementioned steps. In the case of DVDs, the job can be divided among several professionals in order to optimize competences. So, one person may work on transcribing the dialogue with other individuals involved in spotting, working on the translation, adapting the translation into subtitles and finally reviewing. As far as intralingual and interlingual subtitling are concerned, the most obvious difference between these two modalities is, of course, language directionality. Translating from oral into written language is not as problematic and culturally challenging as translating into another language and culture. But, on top of that, the target users are also different: interlingual subtitles are aimed at all possible users of a given language, while intralingual subtitles are specifically aimed at the deaf and hard-of-hearing. In so-called subtitling countries, where subtitling is the main audiovisual translation practice, two versions of the same programme may be provided.

In the case of subtitles for the deaf and hard-of-hearing (SDH) strict conventions must be adhered to. In Italy, for example, conventions at RAI, the state-owned broadcaster, demand different approaches to subtitling depending on whether a programme is originally in Italian, dubbed or whether it is a children's programme.

Which standards do you follow? Are we likely to arrive at European standards for film/TV subtitles?

For Italian TV, intralingual subtitling standards depend on the particular programme. If the programme is originally in Italian, subtitles should be as verbatim as possible so that users have time to lip-read and still refer to the subtitles if they wish to do so. If the source programme is a dubbed one, standards are as follows:

- a maximum of two lines and 36 characters per line;
- three seconds for a full line and five seconds for two full lines (for adults). Four seconds for a full line and eight for two full lines (for children);
- syntax should be as simple as possible and follow the "Subject/Verb/Object" word order;
- semantics should be simplified in order to make subtitles easily comprehensible;
- synchronization must respect shot changes.

The Italian National Institute for the Deaf usually provides feedback to RAI regarding the subtitles they produce.

As regards European standards, the situation is quite complex. Each country has its own tradition and it is difficult to satisfy all users. In the case of intralingual subtitles, for example, it has been suggested that different solutions should be adopted for signing deaf – for whom the written language of the country they live in is a "foreign" language – and for oralist deaf – for whom the spoken and written language of the country they live in is their native tongue. The ongoing *Digital TV for All* project undertaken by a group of European researchers coordinated by Dr Takebumi Itagaki (Brunel University, UK)[1] has concentrated on technical aspects of subtitling (such as character identification, subtitles placement, font and size of letters, etc.) with the aim of reaching a common European standard. Three groups of users were tested for every nation: hearing people, deaf people and hard-of-hearing people. Researchers have concluded that it was not possible to find a common standard for all three groups within the same nation. We can therefore imagine how complicated and perhaps impractical it would be to create common European standards.

1   <http://www.psp-dtv4all.org/> (accessed 28/02/2011).

Certainly, however, if standards were to be introduced, then an independent evaluation committee would be desirable and, perhaps, even essential.

Speaking of the "complexities" of subtitling, one is inclined to regard technical constraints as the biggest issue. Is that true? What would you say are the most challenging aspects of subtitling?

From a technical perspective, almost everything is possible. Constraints are not only due to the limitations of the software used, but to the complexities (linguistic, cultural, sociolinguistic and so on) of the text to be subtitled and to the profile of the end users. Of course, since reading a written text is generally a slower process than listening to the same text produced orally, space constraints are imposed on the subtitler in order to ensure acceptable reading times for the end users. In DVD subtitling, where the possibility to rewind is available and in some subtitling countries, where people have become accustomed to this practice and therefore tend to have a higher reading speed, subtitles can be longer than in TV subtitling and in dubbing countries.

The most challenging task for a subtitler is probably the editing of the source text. Reduction of the source text, one of the techniques most frequently used in subtitling, requires the use of morphological, syntactical and semantic synonyms. Sometimes when a word is altered, the entire sentence must be changed accordingly. It may even be necessary to omit entire semantic units. Then, one must ensure that what follows is coherent with the context. So, in my view, the difficulties are mainly of a linguistic nature and pertain to respecting conventions and not necessarily to technical issues.

What strategies are applied to solve cultural issues in dialogues/scenes with strong culture-specific connotations?

These are the most time-consuming elements to translate, along with technical terminology. Regrettably, one does not always have a file with the transcription of the dialogue, so one must rely on one's own understanding of the audio, where sound may be muffled, disturbed etc. When working from English or other polycentric languages like French or Spanish, terminology can be composed of terms which are specific to linguistically "peripheral" cultures like the Spanish-speaking Caribbean, the French-speaking sub-Saharan, or the English-speaking Oceanic ones. Researching these terms can be time-consuming and time is a luxury the subtitler does not often enjoy. In the case of interlingual subtitles, if an exact or adequate linguistic equivalent cannot be found, then different solutions are possible such as direct or acclimatized loan, calque, hyperonymy, or hyponymy.

As regards technical or specific terminology one must assess the relevance of the term in question, i.e. if the term appears frequently or just once. If it is used sporadically it may be possible to omit it. Specialist terms often appear in documentaries but also in films and TV series which take place in a specialized setting. If, in a TV series located at the ironmonger's a character requests "steel butt hinges" the solutions may vary depending on whether the object is seen on screen or whether it occupies a minor role. If it is not seen, the subtitler may opt for an easy solution, like utilizing a near-synonym, a hyperonym or a hyponym. But if the character insists that he wants "steel butt hinges" and not "steel blackflap hinges" and the two types of hinges are shown, the subtitler cannot avoid terminological research in order to find the exact translation. This is very time-consuming and can pose problems for those subtitlers who are paid per minute of video or per subtitle and not for the time spent on researching and subtitling a programme.

Has subtitling affected or influenced the way you translate written texts?

Yes. Subtitling and the compression involved in the process due to time and space constraints have led me to think in terms of communication. When translating written texts, I was frequently tempted to think in terms of language pairs. However, when translating specialized texts, where the main aim is not linguistic equivalence, but the efficiency of the target text in the communicational setting where it is to be used, I realized that a different approach to translation was necessary and automatisms acquired during subtitling not only assisted me in finding the most legible alternative among different options, but it also helped me to work more efficiently.

Another advantage I derived from subtitling was the overall sense of coherence and cohesion of the target text. When subtitling, you must ensure that what you write is immediately understandable in the context of what comes before. This is very useful for translating texts that are not written by professional writers but by people specialized in other fields.

In your experience, what are the mistakes an inexperienced subtitler is most likely to make?

First of all, conventions and guidelines are so numerous that what for some are mistakes for others are the rule. In general I find that inexperienced subtitlers tend to approach subtitling as an exercise of literal translation. In particular they do not realize that their text is going to be read as a transient text and translate all aspects of the source text, features of orality included, without acknowledging reading time.

Another common error is the lack of cohesion. In oral communication cohesion is possible because of paralinguistic information (intonation, intention, pauses, prosody, body language, etc.). If you transcribe or translate a text which relies on a lot of paralinguistic information or includes repetitions, incoherent syntax and interrupted sentences and so on, the transcribed or translated text runs the risk of being incomprehensible.

Another common error I have encountered is the obsessive requirement for "close" translations. Let us take taboo words, for example. Translating them for interlingual subtitles is very complex. Firstly, expressions using taboo words are culture-specific and only work in the geographical area in which they are used. Also, an exact equivalent can prove difficult to find and to use because the semiosphere is rarely the same and because the occurrence of taboo or other expletives in oral language is generally more acceptable than in a written text. So the tendency to translate everything whilst remaining as faithful as possible to the source text can occasionally be problematic.

A number of third level institutions across Europe offer postgraduate qualifications in subtitling. What professional environment are these postgraduate students likely to find once they enter the job market?

The audiovisual world is changing rapidly and more and more audiovisual products are available and must be subtitled. This means that there is potentially a lot of work for new graduates. However, the problem is how well paid the job will be. In addition, fansubbing is rapidly gaining momentum and its quality can be quite good. An increasing number of people speak at least two languages so it is difficult to anticipate what kind of market these students will find and how much they will earn in the future as compared to subtitlers today. Regarding the interlingual subtitling of film productions one would hope that production and distribution companies will take more interest in this form of audiovisual translation and place a higher value on the considerable work subtitlers do in order for their products to be marketed globally.

Notes on Contributors

EDUARD BARTOLL is an audiovisual translator and has subtitled more than 500 films. He also translates plays. Among the books he has translated: *Die Glücksformel* (S. Klein), *Schweyk* (B. Brecht), *Via Dolorosa* (D. Hare), *Creeps* (L. Hübner), *Der Hässliche* (M. von Mayenburg), *Aussetzer* (L. Hübner), *Täter* (T. Jonigk), *Troilus and Cressid, Macbeth* (W. Shakespeare), *A Disappearing Number* (S. McBurney), *Eurydice* (S. Ruhl). He works at University Pompeu Fabra, in Barcelona, as a lecturer in translation and at the Master in Audiovisual Translation, at the Universitat Autònoma de Barcelona. His PhD on Subtitling will be published in Catalan. Among his articles: Position of subtitles for the deaf and hard of hearing (2010), Learning to subtitle online: Learning environment exercises and evaluation (2008), Subtitling Multilingual Films (2006), Parameters for the classification of subtitles (2004). He is also a member of the Transmedia Catalonia research group.

ŁUKASZ BOGUCKI is Head of the Department of Translation Theory and Practice at Lódz University. His publications include three monographs and over twenty articles on translation, especially audiovisual and computer-assisted translation. He has also co-edited a volume on audiovisual translation. He is a member of the editorial board of *The Journal of Specialised Translation*. For the past sixteen years, he has taught translation at various universities in Europe (including institutions in London, Dublin, Munich, Falun, Porto, Leiria, Tampere, Leuven, Bamberg and Poland). He has organized five international translation conferences. He is a freelancer, translating mostly academic articles from and into Polish.

CLAUDIA BORGHETTI is an Arts graduate of Bologna in 2004. In 2008, she completed her PhD at the National University of Ireland, Galway with a dissertation on intercultural foreign language education. While at the University of Galway, she held the position of Foreign Language Assistant in the Italian Department during the academic years 2005–7. She is currently a researcher at the Department of Modern Foreign Languages and Literatures at the University of Bologna, where she is researching corpus linguistics and foreign language teaching. She also works as a teacher trainer and teaches Italian as a second language to different target students (migrants, university and opera students). Among her main research interests: teaching Italian as a foreign/second language, intercultural education and corpus linguistics in foreign language teaching.

MARCELLA DE MARCO has a degree in Foreign Languages and Literatures from the University of Bari (Italy) and a PhD in Translation and Interpreting from the University of Vic (Spain). She is a Senior Lecturer in Applied Translation Studies at London Metropolitan University and has published various articles on translation and Hispanic philology. Her main academic interests are related to Audiovisual Translation and Gender Studies. Publications: Gender portrayal in dubbed and subtitled comedies. (2009); Audiovisual translation from a gender perspective (2006); Multiple portrayals of gender in cinematographic and audiovisual translation discourse (2006); *Deseo masculino y deseo femenino en las representaciones fílmicas* (2005); *Tecnicismos y cultismos en el "Lapidario" de Alfonso X el Sabio* (2004).

CARLO EUGENI graduated in Conference Interpreting and Translation at the SSLMIT of the University of Bologna. He has a PhD in English for Special Purposes with a thesis on live subtitling by means of speech recognition technology. He teaches Business French at the University of Perugia and Multimedia Translation and Consecutive Interpreting at the University of Macerata. He is the author of several publications in English, French and Italian on respeaking and related aspects (mainly professional and didactic), the organizer of the triennial international seminar on real-time intralingual subtitling, and member of the editorial board of the *The Sign Language Translator and Interpreter* journal. As a freelance subtitler he produces pre-recorded subtitles for RAI teletext and live subtitles for several associations for the deaf. As a freelance trainer he prepares university students and professionals alike for the use of speech recognition technology for subtitling for the deaf and the hard-of-hearing.

MARIA FOUNTANA has a background in education and ICT, a BA in Philosophy, Education and Psychology from the University of Athens, Greece (1999) and an MA in ICT from the University of London (2001). She is currently a PhD candidate in the area of educational technology at the University of Athens. Her research interests include innovation in education related to mobile learning, serious games design and communities of practice. She has been actively involved in several National and European projects as a member of the research group of the Educational Technology Lab since October 2001 and as a member of the RACTI / Educational Technology sector since October 2003. Among her publications: The English Language without (the Physical Presence of the) Teacher: Distance Learning in Multigrade Primary Schools (2006); Game Designing and Game Playing: What We Have Learned from the SimSafety project! The Case of Greece (2010).

MARIA FREDDI is Assistant Professor of English language and linguistics at the University of Pavia, Italy, where she currently teaches courses on English grammar, text and corpus linguistics. She holds a PhD from the Catholic University, Milan, on rhetoric of science and a diploma in music (piano) from Bologna Conservatoire. Her research interests include ESP, in particular the discourse of science and technology, descriptive grammars in an EFL context and corpus linguistics also applied to translation studies. For the past five years she has been involved in a research project on audiovisual translation aimed at designing a computer-readable parallel corpus of British and American movies and their dubbed Italian versions. This research has been published in a collected volume she co-edited with the project's principal investigator, Maria Pavesi, entitled *Analysing Audiovisual Dialogue. Linguistic and Translational Insights* (2009).

ELISA GHIA graduated cum laude in Theoretical and Applied Linguistics from the University of Pavia in 2007, with a dissertation on the effects of exposure to subtitled films on the acquisition of foreign language syntax.

In 2007, she was awarded a scholarship for a doctorate in Linguistics at the same university. Her research deals with the relationship between subtitle translation and second language acquisition. She has spent research periods at the University of Turku, the Katholieke Universiteit Leuven and Michigan State University. At the University of Pavia, she is currently part of an international research project on audiovisual dialogue, translation and language acquisition. She has been English teaching assistant at the University of Pavia and has undertaken didactic activity on audiovisual translation, second language acquisition and research methodology. She has published in the area of language learning and audiovisual translation and has participated in international conferences on translation and comparative linguistics.

LAURA INCALCATERRA MCLOUGHLIN, PhD, is a lecturer at the National University of Ireland, Galway, and also co-director of the MA in Advanced Language Skills, where she teaches Italian language (including Italian for special purposes) and translation. She has published widely on language teaching methodology, language and new technologies and subtitling in language teaching and translators' training. She has presented numerous papers at many international conferences.

JENNIFER LERTOLA is a PhD candidate (Galway Doctoral Research Scholar) in Italian Studies at the National University of Ireland, Galway. She holds a BA in Foreign Languages and Cultures (English and Spanish) from the Università degli Studi di Genova, Italy, and an MA in Teaching Italian as a Foreign Language (MASTER DITALS) from the Universtità per Stranieri di Siena, Italy. Her research interests are audiovisual translation and second language acquisition. Her doctoral research on the effect of subtitling practice on language acquisition in the foreign language class is supervised by Dr Laura Incalcaterra McLoughlin.

SILVIA LURAGHI is Associate Professor of Comparative and General Linguistics at the University of Pavia. She is a specialist in Greek and Latin linguistics, Anatolian, and Indo-European linguistics. Her main research interests concern syntactic and semantic change in the framework of functional-typological and cognitive linguistics. Her published work includes 12 books (e.g. *On the Meaning of Cases and Adpositions*, 2003, *Linguistique historique et indoeuropéenne*, 2010) and numerous papers in refereed journals, such as *Linguistics, Studies in Language* and *Diachronica*. She maintains a parallel vocation in opera criticism and collaborates with leading magazines in the field, such as *Opera News* and *Classic Voice*.

EITHNE O'CONNELL is Senior Lecturer in Translation Studies in SALIS (School of Applied Language and Intercultural Studies) and a member of CTTS (the Centre for Translation and Textual Studies) at Dublin City University, Ireland. She pioneered the first undergraduate and graduate modules in Audiovisual Translation in Ireland and has published widely on subtitling and dubbing training and practice, with particular reference to minority languages, especially Irish, and children. A qualified subtitler herself, she has acted as consultant to the national Irish television broadcasters, RTÉ and the Irish language TV station, TnaG/TG4. She has been twice Chairperson of the MA in Translation Studies at DCU, which recently became a member of the European Masters in Translation (EMT) network. In 2003, she published *Minority Language Dubbing for Children* and in 2008, she co-edited a collection of bilingual essays on Irish language television entitled *TG4@10: Deich mBliana de TG4 /Ten Years of TG4* (Cló Iar-Chonnachta). She is a founder member of ITIA (Irish Translators' and Interpreters' Association) and ESIST (European Association for Studies in Screen Translation).

ELISA PEREGO is a tenured research fellow in English Language and Linguistics at the University of Trieste, where she commenced work and joined the Department of Language, Translation and Interpreting Studies in 2006. Prior to coming to Trieste, she studied at the University of Pavia, where she graduated with merit in Foreign Languages (English and Hungarian) and was awarded a PhD in Linguistics (2004). Her research interests and publications lie mainly in the field of audiovisual translation and include subtitle usability, subtitled films and cognitive processes, film language and audiovisual text analysis, and the perception and processing of subtitled versus dubbed audiovisual texts.

LUPE ROMERO has a PhD in Theory of Translation from the Universitat Autònoma de Barcelona (UAB), where she is a lecturer in Italian language at the Faculty of Translation and Interpreting. She has taught several courses on subtitling at the Universidade Federal de Minas Gerais (Brazil) and has also worked as a professional translator; she has translated more than 25 books and is co-author of a bilingual dictionary (Italian–Spanish). She is a member of PACTE research group, which is highly renowned in the area of translation competence acquisition processes and evaluation, and recently she has been involved in a European research project on Learning via Subtitling (LeViS). Her main areas of research are Audiovisual Translation, Translation Didactics and Translation Competence Acquisition. She has presented her work at many international conferences and published in several international translation journals.

STAVROULA SOKOLI has a BA in English Language and Literature from the Aristotle University of Thessaloniki, Greece, and an MA in Translation Theory from the Universitat Autonoma de Barcelona. Her PhD thesis is on subtitling norms and practices in Greece and Spain. She has taught on the undergraduate course of Hispanic Language and Civilization at the Hellenic Open University and at postgraduate level "Tradumatica: Translation and Localization" at the Universitat Autònoma de Barcelona. She has coordinated the EU-funded project Learning via Subtitling (Socrates/Lingua II, 2006–8) and has over 20 publications and papers in conferences on audiovisual translation, subtitling and language learning, including: Omisión y distribución de subtítulos en España y Grecia: Cómo y por qué (2005); Temas de investigación en traducción audiovisual: La definición del texto audiovisual (2005), and Subtitling Norms in Greece and Spain (2009).

NOA TALAVÁN ZANÓN is junior lecturer in the Foreign Languages Department at the Universidad Nacional de Education a Distancia (UNED), Spain. She graduated in English Philology (Universidad Complutense de Madrid) as well as in Translation and Interpreting (Universidad de Vic) and then obtained a PhD in English Philology from UNED. She has conducted extensive research on audiovisual translation and FLE, as well as in the use of ICT in English for Professional Purposes. She is a certified translator (English–Spanish) and currently the academic coordinator of English C1 at the Centro Universitario de Idiomas a Distancia (Open University Language Centre), Spain.

PATRICK ZABALBEASCOA, born in London in 1961, has lived in Spain since 1971. He completed his PhD in 1993, on a theoretical model for translation based on the variability of factors (namely, priorities and restrictions) for each new translation project. He has further developed these findings and their implications, particularly applied to the translation of humour, metaphors and audiovisuals, both separately and combined. Since 1994 he has lectured in translation theory and practice at the University Pompeu Fabra in Barcelona, Spain. He has contributed towards promoting audiovisual translation studies in Spain through research projects, organizing conferences, founding associations, and reading papers at home and abroad in specialized courses, seminars, and conferences, and through his numerous publications, including: *Translating Audiovisual Screen Irony* (2003) and *The Nature of the Audiovisual Text and its Parameters* (2008).

Index of Names

Index of Terms

New Trends in Translation Studies

In today's globalised society, translation and interpreting are gaining visibility and relevance as a means to foster communication and dialogue in increasingly multicultural and multilingual environments. Practised since time immemorial, both activities have become more complex and multifaceted in recent decades, intersecting with many other disciplines. New Trends in Translation Studies is an international series with the main objectives of promoting the scholarly study of translation and interpreting and of functioning as a forum for the translation and interpreting research community.

This series publishes research on subjects related to multimedia translation and interpreting, in their various social roles. It is primarily intended to engage with contemporary issues surrounding the new multidimensional environments in which translation is flourishing, such as audiovisual media, the internet and emerging new media and technologies. It sets out to reflect new trends in research and in the profession, to encourage flexible methodologies and to promote interdisciplinary research ranging from the theoretical to the practical and from the applied to the pedagogical.

New Trends in Translation Studies publishes translation- and interpreting-oriented books that present high-quality scholarship in an accessible, reader-friendly manner. The series embraces a wide range of publications – monographs, edited volumes, conference proceedings and translations of works in translation studies which do not exist in English. The editor, Dr Jorge Díaz Cintas, welcomes proposals from all those interested in being involved with the series. The working language of the series is English, although in exceptional circumstances works in other languages can be considered for publication. Proposals dealing with specialised translation, translation tools and technology, audiovisual translation and the field of accessibility to the media are particularly welcomed.